Healing With Red Light Therapy

A Revolutionary Approach to Pain Relief, Fat Loss, and Anti-Aging

Dr. Steve H. G. Godson

Healing With Red Light Therapy

Copyright © 2024 by Dr. Steve H. G. Godson

All Rights Reserved.
No part of this book may be used or reproduced by any means, graphic, electronic, or mechanical, including photocopying, recording, taping, or by any information storage retrieval system without the written permission of the publisher.

TABLE OF CONTENTS

Introduction to Red Light Therapy 9
    What Is Red Light Therapy? 9
    The History and Evolution of Light-Based Healing 11
    How Red Light Therapy Works at the Cellular Level 13
    Why Light Therapy Is a Game-Changer in Modern Medicine 16

The Science Behind Red Light Therapy 20
    Understanding the Role of Mitochondria in Cellular Health 21
    How Red and Near-Infrared Light Affect Cellular Function 23
    An Overview of Key Clinical Studies on Red Light Therapy 27
    Debunking Common Myths and Misconceptions 29

Core Benefits of Red Light Therapy 34
    Anti-Aging and Skin Rejuvenation 34
    Pain Relief and Accelerated Healing 37
    Energy Boosting and Fatigue Reduction 40

- Muscle Recovery and Performance Enhancement.................................43
- Mental Clarity, Focus, and Brain Health......46

Red Light Therapy for Skin Health...........................49
- How Red Light Therapy Reduces Wrinkles and Fine Lines............................. 50
- Treatment for Acne, Scars, and Pigmentation Issues...52
- Reversing Signs of Aging: Elasticity, Collagen Production, and Glow.................. 55
- Managing Skin Conditions: Psoriasis, Eczema, and Rosacea...............................58

Enhancing Physical Fitness and Muscle Recovery with Red Light Therapy...62
- Red Light Therapy for Post-Workout Recovery...63
- Increasing Strength and Endurance with Light Therapy... 65
- Preventing and Healing Sports Injuries.......68
- Reducing Inflammation and Muscle Soreness 71

Red Light Therapy for Weight Loss and Metabolism.. 75
- How Red Light Therapy Affects Fat Cells and Metabolism...76
- Combating Obesity: Benefits for Fat Reduction and Toning................................ 79
- Integrating Red Light Therapy with a Healthy Diet and Exercise...83
- Real-Life Success Stories on Fat Loss with Red Light Therapy...................................... 86

Improving Mental Health and Cognitive Function with Red Light Therapy..................90
    Red Light Therapy for Stress and Anxiety Reduction..................91
    Enhancing Memory, Focus, and Mental Clarity..................94
    Supporting Brain Health: Neuroprotective Effects..................97
    Treating Depression and Mood Disorders with Light Therapy..................100

Pain Management and Wound Healing with Red Light Therapy..................104
    How Red Light Therapy Alleviates Chronic Pain..................105
    Targeting Inflammation for Faster Healing 108
    Accelerating Recovery from Injuries and Surgeries..................110
    Success Stories: Using Red Light Therapy for Pain-Free Living..................113

Boosting Immune Function and Overall Health with Red Light Therapy..................117
    Strengthening Immunity with Red Light Therapy..................118
    Reducing Inflammatory Markers and Disease Prevention..................121
    Promoting Better Sleep and Recovery Cycles 124
    Supporting Hormonal Balance and Metabolic Health..................127

Sexual Health and Fertility Enhancement with Red Light Therapy..................131

Benefits for Reproductive Health and Libido... 132

Using Red Light Therapy to Support Fertility.. 135

Improving Circulation and Blood Flow for Sexual Function.. 138

Real-Life Accounts of Red Light Therapy's Impact on Intimacy...................................... 141

Setting Up Red Light Therapy at Home................. 146

Choosing the Right Red Light Therapy Device.. 147

Understanding Light Wavelengths and Intensity Levels.. 152

Placement, Positioning, and Setup Tips... 154

Avoiding Common Mistakes: Safety Tips and Precautions... 157

How to Use Red Light Therapy Effectively............ 160

Step-by-Step Guide to Treatment Timing and Frequency.. 161

Optimal Distance and Duration for Different Conditions... 164

Customised Protocols for Pain, Skin, Fitness, and More.. 168

Tracking Your Progress and Adjusting Your Routine... 172

Maximising Results with Red Light Therapy......... 175

Combining Red Light Therapy with Nutrition and Supplements...................................... 176

Complementary Therapies: Exercise, Meditation, and More............................... 180

Enhancing Results Through Lifestyle

    Adjustments... 185
    Tools for Monitoring Health Improvements..... 188

Exploring Advanced Red Light Therapy Techniques.. 191

    Using Red Light Therapy in Conjunction with Near-Infrared Light...................................... 192

    Combining with Cold Therapy, Sauna, and Other Modalities... 196

    Addressing Complex Health Conditions with Red Light Therapy..................................... 201

    Emerging Trends and Experimental Applications..205

Frequently Asked Questions About Red Light Therapy..208

    Addressing Common Concerns and Safety Queries... 209

    Troubleshooting Tips for Optimal Outcomes... 212

    Understanding Contraindications and When to Consult a Doctor................................... 215

    Myths vs. Facts: Answering Popular Questions...218

Real Stories and Testimonials: The Impact of Red Light Therapy on Lives... 222

    Success Stories from Users Around the World...223

    How Red Light Therapy Has Changed Lives.. 231

    Lessons Learned and Key Takeaways from User Experiences.......................................232

The Future of Red Light Therapy in Medicine....... 235
    New Research and Potential Health Applications 236
    Innovations in Light Therapy Devices and Technologies... 240
    Red Light Therapy in Mainstream and Integrative Medicine.. 243
    How Red Light Therapy Is Shaping the Future of Wellness.. 246

Appendices... 249
    Glossary of Terms and Scientific Concepts.... 249
    Recommended Red Light Therapy Resources and Products..254
        Books... 255
        Devices.. 256
    Key Research Studies and References.......... 258

Healing With Red Light Therapy

Introduction to Red Light Therapy

Red light therapy has emerged as one of the most promising and scientifically supported methods for non-invasive healing and wellness. Leveraging specific wavelengths of light, this therapy has shown impressive effects on cellular health, inflammation reduction, pain relief, skin rejuvenation, and overall vitality.

What Is Red Light Therapy?

Red light therapy (RLT) is a therapeutic technique that uses low-level wavelengths of red and near-infrared light to penetrate the skin and stimulate cellular processes, aiding in healing, repair, and rejuvenation. These specific wavelengths, typically between 600 and 1000 nanometers, can penetrate tissues without causing damage, making them safe and effective for both surface-level and deeper-tissue applications.

In practice, red light therapy involves exposing the body to red or near-infrared light, which can be delivered via LED panels, laser devices, or other specialised equipment. Unlike ultraviolet light, which can cause skin damage, red light has been shown to have a beneficial impact on cell function and overall health. Commonly used in skin clinics, physical therapy offices, and now even at home, red light therapy is employed to manage a range of health issues, including skin conditions, pain, inflammation, and cognitive function.

The History and Evolution of Light-Based Healing

The therapeutic use of light is far from new. Ancient cultures, such as those in Egypt, Greece, and India, recognized sunlight as a vital part of healing. Ancient Egyptians worshipped the sun for its life-giving qualities, while Hippocrates, the Greek "father of medicine," is said to have used sunlight to treat various ailments, a practice known as heliotherapy.

1. **Heliotherapy and Early Light-Based Treatments**

   In the late 19th and early 20th centuries, heliotherapy gained traction as an effective treatment for diseases like tuberculosis and psoriasis. Danish physician Niels Ryberg Finsen received the Nobel Prize in 1903 for his work with light therapy, particularly in treating lupus vulgaris, a skin condition caused by tuberculosis bacteria. He demonstrated that certain wavelengths of light could be focused and applied to kill harmful bacteria and stimulate healing.

2. **Development of Phototherapy**
   As technology advanced, so did the methods for delivering targeted wavelengths of light. In the 1960s, NASA explored light therapy as a way to promote plant growth in space and later found it had therapeutic benefits for wound healing and pain management for astronauts. This marked the beginning of scientific interest in light therapy for human health.
3. **Modern Red Light Therapy**
   By the 1990s, scientists had identified that red and near-infrared wavelengths could penetrate skin and tissue to stimulate mitochondrial function, increase blood circulation, and reduce inflammation. These discoveries led to the development of modern red light therapy devices. Today, red light therapy has evolved into a powerful treatment used worldwide for conditions such as skin rejuvenation, muscle recovery, pain management, and mental health support.

How Red Light Therapy Works at the Cellular Level

Red light therapy operates on a simple yet profound principle: light energy can stimulate cellular activity. At the heart of this process is the mitochondrion, known as the "powerhouse of the cell," responsible for generating energy in the form of adenosine triphosphate (ATP). The specific wavelengths in red and near-infrared light help optimise mitochondrial function, thus impacting overall cellular health.

1. **Absorption of Light by Cytochrome C Oxidase**
   Within the mitochondria lies an enzyme called cytochrome c oxidase, which plays a crucial role in the production of ATP. Red and near-infrared light are absorbed by cytochrome c oxidase, enhancing its activity and enabling cells to produce ATP more efficiently. This increase in cellular energy allows cells to perform their functions better and enhances their ability to repair and rejuvenate.

2. **Reduction of Oxidative Stress and Inflammation**
   Increased ATP production improves cellular resilience, making cells better equipped to handle stress and repair damage. Additionally, red light therapy helps reduce oxidative stress, a harmful process that can cause cellular ageing and inflammation. By reducing oxidative stress and inflammation, red light therapy promotes healing and reduces pain.
3. **Stimulation of Blood Circulation**
   Red light therapy stimulates nitric oxide production, which helps expand blood vessels and improves circulation. Enhanced blood flow brings more oxygen and nutrients to tissues and promotes the removal of waste products. This mechanism is particularly beneficial for healing wounds, reducing muscle soreness, and managing chronic pain.
4. **Modulation of Inflammatory Pathways**
   Red light therapy has been shown to modulate inflammatory pathways, which

can play a significant role in conditions like arthritis, skin disorders, and autoimmune diseases. By reducing inflammation at the cellular level, red light therapy helps mitigate the symptoms of these conditions, promoting a healthier, more balanced body.

Why Light Therapy Is a Game-Changer in Modern Medicine

Red light therapy represents a paradigm shift in the way we approach health and healing. Unlike conventional medicine, which often relies on drugs that come with side effects, light therapy is non-invasive, drug-free, and generally without adverse effects. Its broad range of applications and safety profile makes it an attractive option for those seeking a holistic approach to health.

1. **Safe and Non-Toxic**
   One of the most appealing aspects of red light therapy is its safety. Red light therapy does not rely on pharmaceuticals or invasive procedures, reducing the risk

of side effects or complications. Because it is non-toxic, it is suitable for regular use and can be easily integrated into a wellness routine.

2. **Broad Range of Benefits**
Red light therapy's ability to address a diverse array of health issues is unmatched. From anti-aging and skin health to pain management, cognitive function, and muscle recovery, red light therapy offers a wide range of benefits that appeal to individuals of all ages. Studies have shown its effectiveness in managing conditions like arthritis, depression, chronic pain, and skin damage, making it a versatile and effective therapy.

3. **Emerging Research and Potential Applications**
As more research is conducted, the potential applications of red light therapy continue to expand. Recent studies have explored its use in areas such as brain health, Alzheimer's disease, immune

support, and even fertility. Its ability to enhance mitochondrial function suggests that red light therapy could play a crucial role in managing diseases related to cellular ageing and mitochondrial dysfunction, including metabolic syndrome, cardiovascular disease, and neurodegenerative disorders.

4. **Increasing Accessibility and Ease of Use**
With the advent of user-friendly red light therapy devices, individuals can now access the benefits of this therapy from the comfort of their own homes. The availability of affordable and effective devices has democratised access to red light therapy, empowering individuals to take control of their health in a way that was not possible before.

5. **The Future of Integrative Medicine**
As our understanding of cellular health grows, red light therapy is poised to become a cornerstone of integrative medicine. It aligns well with other holistic therapies, such as diet, exercise, and stress

management, to support optimal health from a cellular level. By addressing the root cause of many conditions—mitochondrial dysfunction—red light therapy holds the potential to revolutionise preventive health and chronic disease management.

The Science Behind Red Light Therapy

Red light therapy (RLT) is more than just a popular wellness trend—it's a scientifically validated approach rooted in cellular biology. By exploring how RLT interacts with cells, particularly mitochondria, we gain a better understanding of its impact on health. This chapter explains the science behind RLT, with an emphasis on mitochondria's role, the specific effects of red and near-infrared light, and key clinical studies. Additionally, it clears up common myths and misconceptions, providing a clear view of the science-backed benefits of red light therapy.

Understanding the Role of Mitochondria in Cellular Health

Mitochondria are often called the "powerhouses" of the cell because they produce adenosine triphosphate (ATP), the energy currency that powers nearly every function in the body. These tiny organelles are responsible for converting nutrients into usable energy through a process called oxidative phosphorylation. Healthy mitochondria are essential for maintaining cellular health, vitality, and overall well-being. They help cells grow, divide, and perform specialised functions, supporting everything from physical energy to cognitive function.

1. **ATP Production and Energy**
   Mitochondria generate ATP, which fuels biochemical processes necessary for cellular activity. ATP is vital for muscle contraction, nerve function, and the maintenance of cell structures. A decrease in mitochondrial efficiency means less

ATP, which can lead to fatigue, ageing, and vulnerability to disease.

2. **Mitochondrial Dysfunction and Aging**
As we age, our mitochondrial function naturally declines, and this reduction in efficiency can have far-reaching effects on health. Mitochondrial dysfunction is linked to several age-related diseases, including neurodegenerative disorders, metabolic syndrome, and cardiovascular disease. Improving mitochondrial function is therefore a key strategy in combating these age-related issues, which is where red light therapy comes into play.

3. **Oxidative Stress and Inflammation**
Mitochondria are also involved in regulating oxidative stress, which is the imbalance between free radicals and antioxidants in the body. When mitochondria are dysfunctional, they can produce excessive free radicals, leading to oxidative damage and inflammation. Chronic inflammation and oxidative stress are major contributors to cellular ageing

and degenerative diseases. Red light therapy, by supporting mitochondrial health, helps reduce these harmful effects.

How Red and Near-Infrared Light Affect Cellular Function

The therapeutic wavelengths in red and near-infrared light penetrate the skin and reach varying depths in tissues. Typically, red light (620-700 nanometers) is absorbed at shallower depths, while near-infrared light (700-1,000 nanometers) penetrates deeper into muscles, joints, and organs. These wavelengths have unique effects on cellular processes, specifically targeting mitochondria to enhance their function.

1. **Photobiomodulation and Cytochrome C Oxidase**
   Red and near-infrared light interact with a critical enzyme in mitochondria called cytochrome c oxidase. This enzyme plays a role in the electron transport chain, which is essential for ATP production. Red light therapy stimulates cytochrome c

oxidase, enhancing its efficiency and promoting increased ATP production. This boost in ATP fuels cellular repair, regeneration, and growth, which can positively affect everything from wound healing to brain function.

2. **Enhanced Cellular Metabolism and Healing**

   By improving mitochondrial function, red light therapy supports faster cellular metabolism and enhanced protein synthesis. This means cells can repair themselves more quickly, regenerate tissues more effectively, and support healing processes. For instance, red light therapy can accelerate wound healing, muscle recovery, and skin regeneration by promoting collagen production.

3. **Reduction of Inflammation**

   Red light therapy also helps reduce inflammation at a cellular level by regulating inflammatory cytokines, which are molecules that play a role in immune response. Lowering inflammation is particularly valuable for people with chronic pain conditions, arthritis, and inflammatory skin conditions, such as eczema or psoriasis. The anti-inflammatory effects of RLT are one of the main reasons it has gained popularity as a non-invasive treatment for pain relief and injury recovery.

4. **Increased Blood Circulation**
Another benefit of red light therapy is its ability to stimulate the production of nitric oxide, a molecule that dilates blood vessels and improves blood flow. Better circulation brings more oxygen and nutrients to tissues, aiding in the removal of waste products and promoting quicker recovery. Improved blood flow is especially useful in managing conditions like muscle soreness, arthritis, and certain circulatory disorders.

An Overview of Key Clinical Studies on Red Light Therapy

Scientific research on red light therapy has increased substantially in recent years, with numerous clinical studies validating its benefits for a variety of health conditions. Here is a summary of some landmark studies that have shaped our understanding of red light therapy's therapeutic potential.

1. **Skin Rejuvenation and Anti-Aging**
   A clinical study published in *Photomedicine and Laser Surgery* demonstrated that red light therapy could significantly improve skin texture, reduce fine lines, and enhance skin tone. The study found that RLT promotes collagen production, leading to firmer and more youthful skin. This research has led to widespread use of RLT in dermatology for non-invasive skin rejuvenation.
2. **Pain Management and Inflammation Reduction**
   Research published in *The Lancet* found that red light therapy effectively reduced pain and inflammation in patients with

chronic joint disorders, such as arthritis. The anti-inflammatory properties of RLT have since been utilised in sports medicine and physical therapy to treat injuries, chronic pain conditions, and postoperative recovery.

3. **Muscle Recovery and Athletic Performance**

   A study conducted by NASA in collaboration with the University of Alabama showed that near-infrared light helped enhance muscle recovery and reduced pain in astronauts. Later studies confirmed similar results in athletes, with red light therapy reducing muscle soreness and accelerating recovery times. As a result, RLT has become popular among athletes looking for natural methods to improve recovery and enhance performance.

4. **Cognitive Function and Brain Health**

   Several studies have explored the use of red light therapy for cognitive function and brain health, particularly in the context of neurodegenerative diseases. Research published in *Photobiomodulation, Photomedicine, and Laser Surgery* showed that near-infrared light can improve cognitive function and reduce symptoms of depression and anxiety by promoting brain cell function and reducing inflammation.

Debunking Common Myths and Misconceptions

Despite its scientifically supported benefits, red light therapy is sometimes surrounded by myths and misconceptions. Let's address and debunk some of the most common ones to clarify what RLT can and cannot do.

1. **Myth: Red Light Therapy is a "Miracle Cure" for All Health Issues**
   Reality:
   While red light therapy has impressive therapeutic benefits, it is not a cure-all. It can significantly improve conditions related to pain, skin health, inflammation,

and mitochondrial function, but it is most effective when used as part of a holistic approach to health. RLT should complement, not replace, other healthy lifestyle practices, such as a balanced diet, exercise, and medical treatment when necessary.

2. **Myth: Any Red Light Will Work for Therapy**
   Reality:
   Not all red lights have therapeutic benefits. For RLT to be effective, it must emit light at specific wavelengths (typically between 600 and 1,000 nanometers). Common red bulbs do not provide the right intensity or wavelength for cellular penetration and do not stimulate mitochondrial function. Certified RLT devices are specially designed for therapeutic use, delivering precise wavelengths for effective results.

3. **Myth: Red Light Therapy is Dangerous Due to Radiation Exposure**
   Reality:

Red light therapy does not use ionising radiation, which can be harmful. Instead, it utilises non-ionizing, low-level light wavelengths that are safe for therapeutic applications. Studies have demonstrated that red and near-infrared light therapy, when used according to guidelines, is safe for long-term use and has no toxic effects on cells or tissues.

4. **Myth: Red Light Therapy Only Benefits Skin and Beauty Applications Reality:**

   While RLT is widely recognized for its benefits in skin health, its applications extend far beyond cosmetic use. Clinical studies have shown its effectiveness in reducing chronic pain, improving brain function, enhancing athletic recovery, and even boosting immune health. Red light therapy can target deep tissues and organs, making it a versatile tool for health and wellness.

5. **Myth: Results are Immediate with One Treatment**

Reality:
While some users may feel a slight improvement after a single session, red light therapy typically requires consistent use over time to achieve optimal results. Most conditions benefit from a routine application of red light therapy for several weeks, if not months, to see sustained improvements.

Core Benefits of Red Light Therapy

Red light therapy (RLT) is a versatile, non-invasive treatment that provides a range of health benefits by harnessing specific wavelengths of red and near-infrared light. These wavelengths penetrate the skin and affect cells at the mitochondrial level, promoting energy production, cellular repair, and overall wellness.

Anti-Aging and Skin Rejuvenation

One of the most popular uses for red light therapy is in the realm of anti-aging and skin rejuvenation. With increasing demand for non-invasive solutions to combat signs of ageing, RLT has become a favoured approach for individuals seeking to improve skin health, reduce wrinkles, and achieve a youthful glow.

1. **Collagen Production and Elasticity**
   Collagen is a protein essential for maintaining the skin's structure, elasticity, and firmness. As we age, collagen production declines, leading to wrinkles and sagging skin. Red light therapy stimulates fibroblasts—cells responsible for producing collagen—thereby promoting natural collagen production. This increase in collagen helps to smooth fine lines, firm the skin, and improve its overall elasticity, giving a rejuvenated and youthful appearance.
2. **Reduction of Fine Lines and Wrinkles**
   RLT's impact on collagen also directly contributes to the reduction of wrinkles.

Clinical studies have shown that red light therapy can diminish fine lines, crow's feet, and other signs of ageing by thickening the skin and improving its texture. This effect is non-invasive, making it a desirable alternative to surgical procedures or injections.

3. **Improved Skin Tone and Texture**
Red light therapy improves skin tone by enhancing cellular turnover and reducing inflammation. This can be especially beneficial for those with sun-damaged skin, hyperpigmentation, or conditions like acne and rosacea. By promoting healthy skin cells, RLT helps to even out pigmentation and improve skin texture, leaving the skin brighter and more even.

4. **Reduction in Acne and Scarring**
Red light therapy's anti-inflammatory properties make it effective in managing acne. The light reduces redness, swelling, and inflammation associated with acne, while also accelerating skin healing to minimise the appearance of scars.

Additionally, red light therapy can help regulate sebum production, which is particularly useful for acne-prone individuals.

Pain Relief and Accelerated Healing

Red light therapy has emerged as a valuable tool for managing pain and accelerating the body's natural healing processes. Its ability to penetrate deep into tissues, combined with its non-invasive nature, makes it an appealing alternative for pain relief and injury recovery.

1. **Reduction of Inflammation**
   One of the primary ways RLT helps with pain relief is by reducing inflammation. Chronic inflammation is often the root cause of pain and discomfort in conditions such as arthritis, joint pain, and muscle strain. Red light therapy modulates inflammatory responses by reducing pro-inflammatory cytokines, which are

molecules involved in the body's immune response. This helps relieve pain while facilitating healing.

2. **Enhanced Blood Flow and Circulation**
RLT has been shown to improve blood flow by stimulating the production of nitric oxide, a molecule that dilates blood vessels and improves circulation. Enhanced blood flow delivers oxygen and nutrients to tissues more efficiently and helps remove waste products, which is especially beneficial for individuals with chronic pain or circulatory conditions. Improved circulation also accelerates healing by bringing more resources to injured areas.

3. **Pain Relief for Joints and Muscles**
Studies have shown that red light therapy is effective in managing pain in joints, such as those affected by arthritis or injury. By penetrating deeply into tissues, RLT can alleviate muscle soreness, reduce stiffness, and improve flexibility, making it an ideal therapy for athletes and

individuals with chronic joint conditions. It provides a natural, drug-free alternative for pain management without the side effects of conventional pain medications.

4. **Wound Healing and Tissue Repair**
RLT accelerates wound healing by promoting cellular regeneration and increasing ATP production, which provides cells with the energy they need to repair damaged tissue. This application is particularly valuable for post-surgical recovery, as it can reduce healing time and lower the risk of infection. Additionally, RLT has been shown to be beneficial for conditions like diabetic ulcers and other wounds that are slow to heal.

Energy Boosting and Fatigue Reduction

Fatigue is a common issue that can stem from various factors, including stress, poor sleep, and mitochondrial dysfunction. Red light therapy boosts energy levels by enhancing mitochondrial efficiency and stimulating cellular processes that support overall vitality.

1. **Enhanced Mitochondrial Function**
   The mitochondria play a crucial role in producing energy at the cellular level, and red light therapy has a profound impact on their function. By targeting cytochrome c oxidase, an enzyme in the mitochondrial electron transport chain, RLT helps produce more ATP (adenosine triphosphate), which is essential for cellular energy. This increase in ATP production translates into more energy available for physical and mental activities, combating fatigue.
2. **Improved Sleep and Circadian Rhythm**
   RLT can positively impact sleep by influencing circadian rhythms. Exposure to red and near-infrared light in the morning or early evening can support the body's natural sleep-wake cycle, leading to improved sleep quality and duration. Better sleep contributes to higher energy

levels and a more balanced mood, which can alleviate feelings of fatigue and burnout.

3. **Increased Alertness and Stamina**
Many people report feeling more alert and energised after red light therapy sessions. The combination of increased cellular energy and reduced inflammation leads to improved stamina, allowing individuals to maintain higher levels of physical and mental endurance throughout the day. This can be particularly beneficial for athletes, busy professionals, or anyone experiencing low energy levels.

Muscle Recovery and Performance Enhancement

Athletes and fitness enthusiasts increasingly turn to red light therapy to aid in muscle recovery and performance enhancement. RLT's benefits for muscles include faster recovery, reduced soreness, and improved endurance, making it a valuable tool for those looking to optimise their workouts.

1. **Reduction in Muscle Soreness and Stiffness**
   Red light therapy helps reduce delayed onset muscle soreness (DOMS), a common occurrence after intense physical activity. By increasing blood flow and reducing inflammation, RLT alleviates stiffness and soreness, helping athletes recover more quickly. This is especially beneficial for those in high-intensity training or repetitive sports activities, as it reduces the downtime needed for muscle recovery.

2. **Enhanced Muscle Growth and Strength**
   Studies suggest that RLT can stimulate muscle growth by enhancing mitochondrial efficiency and promoting protein synthesis. By providing cells with more ATP, RLT helps muscles recover faster and strengthens muscle tissue. Some athletes and bodybuilders use RLT as part

of their routine to accelerate muscle growth and optimise strength.

3. **Improved Endurance and Stamina**
Red light therapy can also improve endurance by reducing fatigue in muscle tissues. By boosting mitochondrial function, RLT helps muscles maintain high performance over extended periods, making it easier to sustain physical activity. This increased stamina is beneficial for both athletes and individuals who engage in regular exercise or physically demanding jobs.

4. **Faster Recovery from Injuries**
Red light therapy aids in tissue repair and regeneration, which speeds up recovery from sports-related injuries, strains, and sprains. It reduces downtime by promoting cellular healing processes and improving circulation, making it an ideal recovery tool for both amateur and professional athletes.

Mental Clarity, Focus, and Brain Health

The benefits of red light therapy extend beyond physical wellness and include mental clarity, focus, and brain health. Research has shown that near-infrared light, in particular, can penetrate the skull and influence brain function, offering a promising approach to cognitive health and mental performance.

1. **Increased Cognitive Function and Focus**
   By improving mitochondrial function and cellular energy production, red light therapy supports better brain function. Increased ATP in brain cells leads to improved mental clarity, focus, and cognitive performance. Studies have shown that RLT can enhance memory, learning, and executive function, making it beneficial for students, professionals, and older adults alike.
2. **Mood Enhancement and Reduction of Anxiety**
   Red light therapy can have a positive

effect on mood by regulating neurotransmitters and reducing inflammation in the brain. Low-level inflammation is linked to mood disorders, including depression and anxiety, and RLT helps mitigate this by promoting a balanced immune response. This effect can contribute to a calmer mood, better stress management, and a reduction in feelings of anxiety.

3. **Neuroprotection and Brain Health**
   Emerging research suggests that red light therapy may offer neuroprotective effects by reducing oxidative stress and inflammation in brain cells. This is particularly valuable for individuals at risk of neurodegenerative diseases such as Alzheimer's and Parkinson's. By supporting mitochondrial health and cellular resilience, RLT may help preserve cognitive function and slow down the progression of age-related brain conditions.

4. **Enhanced Sleep and Stress Reduction** Improved sleep quality, supported by RLT's impact on circadian rhythms, contributes to better mental health and focus. The calming effects of red light therapy also reduce stress by promoting relaxation and supporting a balanced cortisol response. With improved sleep and lower stress levels, individuals experience sharper focus, greater resilience, and better overall brain health.

Red Light Therapy for Skin Health

Red light therapy (RLT) has become one of the most sought-after treatments for various skin issues, including ageing, acne, scars, pigmentation, and chronic skin conditions. Using wavelengths that penetrate deeply into the skin, red light therapy stimulates cellular activity and healing processes, offering a non-invasive solution for achieving clearer, healthier, and younger-looking skin.

How Red Light Therapy Reduces Wrinkles and Fine Lines

One of the most well-known benefits of red light therapy is its ability to reduce wrinkles and fine lines, providing a natural way to achieve youthful skin without surgery or injections.

1. **Stimulating Collagen Production**
   Collagen is the protein responsible for skin's elasticity, structure, and firmness. As we age, collagen production naturally declines, leading to the development of wrinkles, sagging, and fine lines. Red light therapy stimulates fibroblast cells, which are responsible for producing collagen. The wavelengths of red and near-infrared light penetrate the skin layers to reach these cells, promoting collagen synthesis and strengthening the skin's structural integrity. This increase in collagen not only reduces the appearance of wrinkles but also enhances skin texture, making it smoother and firmer.
2. **Promoting Elastin Production**
   Elastin, like collagen, is essential for skin's elasticity. Red light therapy boosts

elastin production, helping the skin regain its natural bounce and resilience. Increased elastin helps to minimise sagging and drooping, making the skin appear plumper and more youthful.

3. **Improving Blood Circulation and Cellular Turnover**

   RLT also improves blood flow to the skin, which delivers oxygen and essential nutrients to skin cells. This enhanced circulation, combined with increased cellular turnover, enables the skin to heal and regenerate faster. This not only helps diminish fine lines but also contributes to a healthy, glowing complexion.

4. **Reduction of Crow's Feet and Other Fine Lines**

   Studies have shown that regular use of red light therapy can significantly reduce common areas where fine lines and wrinkles appear, such as around the eyes, mouth, and forehead. RLT's effect on collagen and elastin production helps smooth these areas, giving the face a more relaxed and youthful appearance.

Treatment for Acne, Scars, and Pigmentation Issues

Acne, scarring, and pigmentation concerns can be difficult to treat with traditional skincare products. Red light therapy offers a safe, drug-free solution by targeting inflammation, bacteria, and pigmentation at the cellular level.

1. **Managing Acne and Reducing Bacteria**
   Acne is often caused by bacteria and inflammation within the skin. Red light therapy has anti-inflammatory properties that reduce swelling and redness associated with acne. Additionally, it can help reduce acne-causing bacteria by enhancing the immune response of skin cells, creating an environment less conducive to bacterial growth. The result

is fewer breakouts and faster healing times for active acne.

2. **Reducing Acne Scarring**

   One of the most challenging aspects of acne is the scarring that often follows. Red light therapy promotes cellular regeneration and collagen production, which can reduce the visibility of scars. By increasing collagen in the affected areas, RLT helps to smooth and repair damaged skin, minimising the appearance of acne scars over time. Regular red light sessions can significantly improve skin texture and even out skin tone in areas with acne scarring.

3. **Addressing Hyperpigmentation and Sun Damage**

   Hyperpigmentation, whether caused by sun damage, hormonal changes, or post-inflammatory marks from acne, can be improved with red light therapy. RLT promotes an even skin tone by accelerating the turnover of pigmented cells and supporting healthier cellular functions. Sun-damaged skin can particularly benefit from RLT, as the light waves help to repair and restore damaged tissue, making it an effective treatment for age spots, sunspots, and melasma.

4. **Evening Out Skin Tone and Texture**
With regular use, red light therapy helps to balance pigmentation, resulting in a more uniform skin tone. It also aids in smoothing out rough skin texture by encouraging cellular repair and improving the skin's overall structure. These effects contribute to a smoother, clearer complexion with a noticeable reduction in spots and uneven areas.

Reversing Signs of Aging: Elasticity, Collagen Production, and Glow

Ageing affects skin in multiple ways, including loss of elasticity, reduced collagen, and diminished radiance. Red light therapy offers a powerful way to combat these signs of ageing by targeting the skin's fundamental processes.

1. **Improving Skin Elasticity**
   Elasticity decreases as skin ages, leading to sagging and drooping, particularly around the jawline, cheeks, and neck. By stimulating elastin fibres, RLT helps restore skin elasticity, allowing the skin to "snap back" more effectively. This improvement in elasticity is one of the most noticeable effects, as it gives the skin a lifted and tightened appearance, restoring a youthful contour to the face and neck.
2. **Increasing Collagen Density**
   The loss of collagen is a primary factor in the visible ageing process. Red light therapy effectively stimulates collagen production, helping to "fill in" areas that may have thinned due to age. This increase in collagen density helps maintain a fuller, firmer appearance,

reducing the appearance of fine lines, wrinkles, and hollow areas.

3. **Enhancing Natural Radiance and Glow**
As red light therapy improves cellular function and circulation, it naturally enhances the skin's radiance. Improved blood flow provides a healthy, rosy glow to the skin, making it look fresher and more vibrant. This effect is particularly valuable for individuals with dull or tired-looking skin, as it revives the complexion and gives it a youthful, revitalised appearance.

4. **Minimising Age Spots and Discoloration**
Age spots and discoloration caused by sun exposure or hormonal changes can be effectively treated with red light therapy. RLT accelerates cellular repair, helping to reduce the appearance of these spots over time. As a result, the skin becomes more even-toned, contributing to a younger-looking complexion.

Managing Skin Conditions: Psoriasis, Eczema, and Rosacea

Chronic skin conditions such as psoriasis, eczema, and rosacea can be difficult to manage and are often associated with inflammation, irritation, and discomfort. Red light therapy offers a non-invasive approach to relieve symptoms and improve skin health in those with these conditions.

1. **Psoriasis**
   Psoriasis is an autoimmune condition characterised by rapid skin cell turnover, leading to scaly, inflamed patches of skin. Red light therapy has shown promise in reducing the frequency and severity of psoriasis flare-ups. The anti-inflammatory effects of RLT help to calm the immune response, reducing redness, scaling, and itching. By promoting cellular repair and reducing inflammation, red light therapy can provide relief from psoriasis

symptoms without the side effects of traditional treatments.

2. **Eczema**

    Eczema, or atopic dermatitis, is another inflammatory skin condition marked by dry, itchy patches of skin that can become red and inflamed. Red light therapy helps manage eczema symptoms by reducing inflammation and promoting moisture retention within the skin. RLT supports the skin's natural barrier function, improving its ability to retain hydration, which can help reduce the frequency and intensity of eczema flare-ups. Its soothing effect makes it a valuable option for individuals with sensitive skin prone to irritation.

3. **Rosacea**

    Rosacea causes redness and visible blood vessels on the skin, typically on the cheeks, nose, and forehead. RLT can help manage rosacea by reducing inflammation and calming overactive blood vessels, which are common in this condition. The gentle light penetrates the skin without causing irritation, making it a suitable option for rosacea patients, who often struggle with treatments that exacerbate their symptoms. With regular sessions, red light therapy can reduce the intensity of redness and flare-ups, providing a long-term solution for rosacea management.

4. **General Benefits for Sensitive Skin**
   For those with sensitive skin, red light therapy provides a non-irritating, non-invasive treatment option. Unlike harsh chemical peels, laser treatments, or prescription creams, RLT is gentle and unlikely to cause additional skin sensitivity or irritation. It enhances the skin's resilience to environmental factors and strengthens its barrier function, making it an effective option for individuals who cannot tolerate traditional treatments.

Enhancing Physical Fitness and Muscle Recovery with Red Light Therapy

Red light therapy (RLT) has become a popular tool among athletes, fitness enthusiasts, and physical therapists for its ability to support physical fitness, accelerate muscle recovery, and reduce injury risk. By harnessing the therapeutic power of specific wavelengths of light, red light therapy penetrates muscles and tissues, targeting cells and enhancing recovery processes. From reducing inflammation and soreness to strengthening muscles and increasing endurance, red light therapy offers a holistic approach to physical fitness and performance enhancement.

Red Light Therapy for Post-Workout Recovery

One of the primary benefits of red light therapy is its role in post-workout recovery. Intense workouts, whether aerobic or anaerobic, cause small tears in muscle fibres, which need to repair and rebuild for strength gains and recovery. Red light therapy speeds up this process, allowing individuals to recover faster and train more consistently.

1. **Reducing Muscle Fatigue**
   During exercise, muscle cells use large amounts of ATP (adenosine triphosphate), which is the energy molecule that powers

cellular functions. High-intensity workouts often deplete ATP reserves, leading to fatigue. Red light therapy stimulates mitochondria, the energy-producing centres of cells, to produce more ATP. This increase in ATP production reduces fatigue, allowing muscles to recover energy levels faster after a workout.

2. **Reducing Lactic Acid Build-Up**
   The buildup of lactic acid in muscles is a common cause of post-exercise discomfort and soreness. Red light therapy promotes circulation, which helps flush out lactic acid more quickly. This improves the body's ability to clear metabolic waste from muscles, reducing delayed-onset muscle soreness (DOMS) and enhancing overall comfort in the days following an intense workout.

3. **Supporting Muscle Tissue Repair and Growth**
   Exercise creates microtears in muscle fibres, and the body's natural repair

process involves rebuilding these fibres stronger than before, a process known as hypertrophy. Red light therapy accelerates tissue repair by enhancing cellular activity and reducing oxidative stress. This makes red light therapy particularly beneficial for athletes and those engaged in regular strength training, as it allows for faster recovery and encourages muscle growth.

Increasing Strength and Endurance with Light Therapy

Red light therapy isn't just beneficial for recovery; it also has potential applications in building strength and increasing endurance. By boosting cellular function and reducing inflammation, RLT helps improve physical performance, enabling individuals to push their limits during workouts.

1. **Increasing ATP Production for Enhanced Stamina**

The mitochondria, known as the "powerhouses" of cells, produce ATP, which fuels muscle contractions during exercise. Red light therapy's ability to stimulate mitochondria to produce more ATP means that muscles have a greater supply of energy to draw upon during activity. This increase in ATP allows for longer, more sustained efforts, improving stamina and endurance over time.

2. **Boosting Muscle Strength**

   Red light therapy stimulates protein synthesis in muscle cells, which plays a key role in muscle growth and strength development. Research has shown that athletes who use red light therapy as part of their training regimen often experience faster strength gains than those who do not. By accelerating muscle protein synthesis, RLT supports gains in strength and power, which are essential for many athletic activities.

3. **Improving Blood Flow and Oxygenation**

Red light therapy improves circulation by stimulating the production of nitric oxide, a molecule that dilates blood vessels and enhances blood flow. Improved circulation delivers oxygen and nutrients to working muscles more effectively, which supports performance and prevents early fatigue. Oxygenated muscles can work harder and longer, allowing athletes to perform better during both endurance and strength-based activities.

Preventing and Healing Sports Injuries

Injuries are an inevitable part of intense physical activity, but red light therapy can help prevent and manage injuries by promoting healing and reducing the risk of re-injury. With its ability to penetrate deeply into tissues, red light therapy offers therapeutic benefits that accelerate tissue repair, reduce inflammation, and restore mobility.

Healing With Red Light Therapy

1. **Accelerating Soft Tissue Repair**
   Sprains, strains, and tears are common injuries among athletes, and these injuries can sideline training for weeks or months. Red light therapy accelerates the healing process by stimulating fibroblasts, the cells responsible for producing collagen, an essential protein for tissue repair. By promoting collagen synthesis, red light therapy helps heal damaged ligaments, tendons, and muscles faster, allowing athletes to return to activity sooner.
2. **Reducing Scar Tissue Formation**
   When an injury heals, the body often creates scar tissue, which can limit mobility and increase the risk of re-injury. Red light therapy minimises scar tissue formation by enhancing the tissue repair process and improving the alignment of collagen fibres as they heal. This results in stronger, more flexible tissue that is less prone to injury and stiffness, making red light therapy an effective solution for long-term injury management.

3. **Preventing Overuse Injuries**
   Overuse injuries, such as tendonitis and stress fractures, are common in athletes who train frequently. By improving blood circulation and promoting recovery between training sessions, red light therapy can help prevent the onset of these injuries. Regular RLT treatments can act as a preventive measure, supporting tissue health and resilience and allowing athletes to maintain consistent training schedules.
4. **Managing Joint Pain and Stiffness**
   Many physical activities place stress on joints, which can lead to pain and stiffness over time. Red light therapy reduces joint inflammation, alleviates pain, and improves joint mobility. This is particularly beneficial for athletes in high-impact sports, as it helps keep joints flexible and reduces the risk of joint-related injuries, making it easier to stay active and train effectively.

Reducing Inflammation and Muscle Soreness

Exercise and physical activity often lead to inflammation and soreness, especially after intense or unaccustomed activity. Red light therapy's anti-inflammatory effects make it an effective tool for managing inflammation, reducing soreness, and promoting a faster recovery.

1. **Inhibiting Inflammatory Pathways**
   Intense exercise triggers an inflammatory response, which can lead to pain, swelling, and stiffness. Red light therapy reduces inflammation by inhibiting inflammatory cytokines, the molecules responsible for promoting inflammation in the body. By reducing cytokine activity, red light therapy helps control inflammation levels, minimising post-exercise discomfort and soreness.
2. **Promoting Muscle Relaxation**
   Tight, sore muscles can limit mobility and interfere with workout performance. Red light therapy promotes muscle relaxation

by increasing blood flow and releasing tension. By relieving muscle stiffness, RLT enables athletes to recover more quickly and return to training with greater ease. The warmth generated by the therapy also provides a soothing effect, further relieving any lingering tightness in muscles.

3. **Preventing Chronic Inflammation in Athletes**
Chronic inflammation can develop in athletes who train consistently without adequate recovery, leading to conditions like tendinitis and muscle fatigue. Red light therapy's ability to control inflammation helps prevent this cycle, promoting healthier muscles and joints. Consistent use of red light therapy aids in managing inflammation over time, supporting tissue health and reducing the risk of chronic injuries.

4. **Enhancing Circulation and Nutrient Delivery**
Red light therapy increases circulation,

which helps deliver essential nutrients to muscles and tissues that need repair. Improved circulation reduces recovery time and supports muscle health by enhancing the body's ability to deliver nutrients and oxygen directly to damaged areas. This benefit makes it especially useful for those who train regularly and need to recover quickly between sessions.

Red Light Therapy for Weight Loss and Metabolism

Red light therapy (RLT) has emerged as an innovative approach to weight loss and metabolic health, drawing interest from researchers, healthcare professionals, and those looking to improve their fitness and overall health. By targeting cellular processes that influence fat cells and energy metabolism, RLT offers a non-invasive, natural solution for enhancing weight loss efforts, improving body composition, and supporting overall metabolic health.

How Red Light Therapy Affects Fat Cells and Metabolism

Red light therapy penetrates the skin and targets adipocytes, the cells responsible for storing fat in the body. It uses specific wavelengths of light, typically in the red and near-infrared spectrum, to stimulate processes within these fat cells and other tissues.

1. **Stimulating Lipolysis (Fat Breakdown)**
   One of the main ways red light therapy promotes fat loss is by stimulating a process known as lipolysis, which breaks down stored fats into free fatty acids and glycerol. When exposed to red light, fat cells release these fatty acids, making them available for the body to use as energy. This helps reduce the volume of fat stored in the body and can support a

gradual decrease in body fat over time. Lipolysis initiated by red light therapy is often referred to as "photobiomodulation," which influences the cell's mitochondrial function, increasing cellular energy and prompting fat cell release.

2. **Enhancing Mitochondrial Function for Increased Energy Production**

   Red light therapy stimulates mitochondria, the energy powerhouses of cells, to produce more ATP (adenosine triphosphate), which is the primary energy currency in the body. This increased ATP production supports higher energy levels, which can lead to greater physical activity, metabolic rate, and calorie expenditure. By helping cells operate more efficiently, RLT may contribute to an enhanced metabolic rate, even in resting states, thereby supporting long-term weight management.

3. **Improving Blood Flow and Oxygen Supply to Tissues**

   Improved circulation is another effect of

red light therapy, as it enhances the production of nitric oxide, a compound that dilates blood vessels and increases blood flow. Better circulation and oxygen delivery mean that muscle tissues are better able to utilise fat as a source of fuel, enhancing the body's ability to burn fat for energy. This is particularly beneficial for individuals engaging in physical activity, as it promotes better endurance and supports fat oxidation during workouts.

4. **Reducing Inflammation and Supporting Hormone Balance**
Chronic inflammation is linked to weight gain and metabolic dysfunction, as it disrupts normal hormonal balance, including insulin and cortisol levels. By reducing inflammation, red light therapy helps restore a healthy balance of these hormones, which play crucial roles in fat storage and breakdown. Balanced insulin levels help prevent fat accumulation, while cortisol reduction can prevent stress-induced weight gain. This makes

RLT a useful tool for managing weight by targeting the underlying metabolic and hormonal imbalances that contribute to obesity.

Combating Obesity: Benefits for Fat Reduction and Toning

In addition to its cellular-level effects, red light therapy has shown promise as a complementary tool in managing obesity, supporting targeted fat reduction, and improving body composition. The therapy can help reshape areas of the body prone to stubborn fat retention, such as the abdomen, thighs, and arms, making it a viable option for those seeking both aesthetic and health-related outcomes.

1. **Targeted Fat Reduction**
   One of the advantages of red light therapy over traditional weight loss methods is its ability to target specific areas. Unlike general weight loss, which may reduce fat

across the body, RLT can concentrate on areas where fat reduction is most desired, such as the waistline or thighs. Research indicates that red light therapy can lead to visible reductions in body circumference when applied to these areas, providing a toning effect that enhances the overall shape of the body.

2. **Improving Skin Tightness and Elasticity**

   When fat cells shrink, they leave behind loose skin in areas where significant fat loss has occurred. Red light therapy supports collagen and elastin production, which helps the skin tighten and maintain its structure. This contributes to a more toned appearance and prevents the sagging that sometimes follows rapid weight loss. By boosting skin elasticity, red light therapy can complement weight loss efforts by ensuring a smoother and firmer result.

3. **Reducing Visceral Fat and Improving Metabolic Health**

Unlike subcutaneous fat, which lies just below the skin, visceral fat surrounds organs and is linked to serious health risks such as cardiovascular disease and diabetes. Studies indicate that red light therapy may help reduce visceral fat by improving insulin sensitivity and decreasing inflammation, both of which are critical factors in visceral fat accumulation. By addressing metabolic dysfunction associated with visceral fat, RLT not only aids in aesthetic body shaping but also promotes long-term health.

4. **Improving Muscle Definition and Toning**

   RLT enhances muscle recovery and growth by increasing ATP production and reducing inflammation in muscle tissues. These benefits can indirectly contribute to weight loss by enabling more effective workouts and promoting muscle development. Increased muscle mass boosts resting metabolic rate, as muscles burn more calories than fat even at rest, creating a sustainable advantage for weight loss and body composition.

Integrating Red Light Therapy with a Healthy Diet and Exercise

While red light therapy can provide significant benefits for weight loss and metabolic health, it is most effective when integrated into a comprehensive wellness plan that includes balanced nutrition and regular physical activity.

1. **Supporting Caloric Deficits and Fat Oxidation**
   Achieving a caloric deficit through diet is fundamental to weight loss. Red light therapy enhances this process by supporting fat oxidation, making it easier for the body to use stored fat as energy. Combined with a diet rich in lean proteins, whole grains, and healthy fats, RLT can

optimise weight loss by encouraging the body to break down fat more efficiently.

2. **Improving Exercise Performance and Recovery**
Regular physical activity is crucial for weight loss and maintenance. Red light therapy can boost performance by enhancing endurance and reducing muscle soreness, allowing individuals to work out more frequently and at higher intensities. The quicker recovery times facilitated by RLT also mean that muscles can repair and grow more efficiently, contributing to a leaner and stronger physique.

3. **Balancing Macronutrients for Optimal Metabolism**
For those integrating red light therapy into a weight loss regimen, maintaining a balanced intake of proteins, fats, and carbohydrates is essential. Protein supports muscle recovery, while healthy fats provide sustained energy for daily activities and workouts. Carbohydrates are necessary for energy but should be

consumed in moderation to avoid insulin spikes. Red light therapy complements these macronutrient strategies by optimising energy production and supporting fat oxidation during and after exercise.

4. **Staying Consistent with RLT and Lifestyle Habits**
Consistency is key to seeing results with red light therapy. Regular sessions, typically a few times a week, allow the body to benefit fully from the therapy's cellular effects. Paired with a steady diet and exercise routine, red light therapy can help individuals stay on track with their weight loss goals and avoid the pitfalls of rapid, unsustainable methods.

Real-Life Success Stories on Fat Loss with Red Light Therapy

Many individuals have experienced significant improvements in their weight loss journeys thanks to red light therapy. Here are some examples of real-life success stories illustrating how RLT has helped people achieve their fat loss and metabolic health goals:

1. **Reduced Body Fat and Inches Lost**
   Numerous users report noticeable reductions in body fat and circumferential measurements after consistent red light therapy sessions. Some individuals have reported losing several inches around their waists, hips, and thighs after a few months of regular treatment, combined with exercise and a balanced diet. These reductions in body fat often correlate with a more toned appearance, providing visible confirmation of RLT's effectiveness.
2. **Enhanced Energy and Stamina**
   Those who struggle with energy levels during weight loss programs often find RLT helpful in overcoming fatigue. Many report that red light therapy boosts their energy, allowing them to engage in more

intense workouts. This increased stamina has led to improved fitness levels, greater calorie expenditure, and accelerated fat loss, reinforcing the synergy between RLT and physical activity.

3. **Improved Skin Texture and Body Contouring**
In addition to fat loss, many individuals experience enhanced skin tone and firmness, especially in areas prone to sagging after weight loss. This is particularly beneficial for those who have achieved significant weight loss and want to improve their skin's appearance. Red light therapy's ability to boost collagen production helps minimise loose skin, providing a smoother, firmer look that complements their new physique.

4. **Success in Combating Stubborn Fat Areas**
Users who struggle with stubborn fat deposits that do not respond well to traditional diet and exercise have found success with red light therapy. Specific

areas like the abdomen, arms, and thighs tend to hold onto fat longer, but with consistent RLT sessions, many users report reduction in these areas, leading to a more balanced and sculpted body shape.

Improving Mental Health and Cognitive Function with Red Light Therapy

Red light therapy (RLT) has demonstrated significant promise in supporting mental health and cognitive function. Its ability to penetrate the skin and affect cellular processes offers a unique approach to managing issues like stress, anxiety, and mood disorders, while also enhancing memory, focus, and overall brain health. This non-invasive therapy uses wavelengths of red and near-infrared (NIR) light to stimulate cellular activity, especially within the mitochondria, and has been shown to support mental clarity and neuroprotection.

Red Light Therapy for Stress and Anxiety Reduction

Stress and anxiety are two of the most prevalent mental health concerns globally, often leading to a host of physical and mental health issues. Red light therapy's potential to help alleviate these conditions lies in its ability to reduce inflammation, regulate neurotransmitter activity, and promote relaxation.

1. **Reducing Inflammation and Cortisol Levels**
   Stress and anxiety are closely linked to inflammation and high cortisol levels, which create a state of chronic stress in the body. RLT has been shown to reduce inflammation through its effects on

cellular mitochondria, which can lower the body's stress response. Reduced inflammation can improve mental well-being by creating a calmer internal environment and reducing the physical symptoms associated with stress. Additionally, some studies suggest that red light therapy can help regulate cortisol, the body's primary stress hormone, which plays a significant role in managing the physical and mental impact of stress.

2. **Regulating Neurotransmitters for Calming Effects**

    Red light therapy may influence key neurotransmitters involved in stress response and mood regulation, such as serotonin and dopamine. By stimulating the brain's neural circuits, red light can help increase the release of these neurotransmitters, creating a calming effect and contributing to a more balanced mood. These biochemical changes encourage relaxation and reduce anxiety symptoms, making RLT a useful tool for managing both situational and chronic stress.

3. **Promoting Deep Relaxation and Better Sleep**
   RLT may also help improve sleep quality, which is crucial for managing anxiety and stress. Exposure to RLT can promote the release of melatonin, a hormone that regulates sleep. Improved sleep quality helps restore energy, lower anxiety levels, and improve the body's ability to cope with stress. Many individuals who use RLT report better sleep, which supports a positive feedback loop, as better sleep can directly contribute to decreased stress and anxiety.

Enhancing Memory, Focus, and Mental Clarity

Cognitive functions such as memory, focus, and mental clarity are influenced by the brain's ability to efficiently produce energy, maintain neuronal health, and repair itself. Red light therapy has been shown to impact these factors positively, promoting a state of enhanced cognitive function.

1. **Boosting Cellular Energy Production in Neurons**
   The mitochondria within brain cells play a key role in cognitive health. RLT stimulates the mitochondria, enhancing ATP (adenosine triphosphate) production and increasing energy availability in the brain. This boost in energy allows neurons to function more effectively, enhancing cognitive processes like memory recall, attention span, and problem-solving abilities. Many users report improved focus and mental clarity following regular RLT sessions, which they attribute to the increased energy in their brain cells.
2. **Improving Blood Flow to the Brain**
   Red light therapy stimulates the production of nitric oxide, a compound

that relaxes blood vessels and improves blood flow. Increased circulation delivers more oxygen and nutrients to the brain, which are essential for maintaining cognitive health. Better blood flow also aids in the removal of toxins, reducing oxidative stress and improving overall brain function. This improvement can help individuals experience sharper focus, faster processing speeds, and enhanced memory retention.

3. **Supporting Neurogenesis and Synaptic Plasticity**

    Some studies indicate that red light therapy may promote neurogenesis, the process by which new neurons are formed in the brain. RLT also supports synaptic plasticity, the ability of the brain to reorganise itself and create new connections between neurons. These processes are essential for memory formation, learning, and adaptation. By supporting neurogenesis and plasticity, RLT can enhance learning abilities, improve long-term memory retention, and help the brain recover from mental fatigue more effectively.

Supporting Brain Health: Neuroprotective Effects

Protecting the brain from degeneration and cognitive decline is a growing concern, particularly with ageing populations and the rising incidence of neurodegenerative conditions like Alzheimer's and Parkinson's. Red light therapy has shown potential neuroprotective effects, providing a proactive approach to maintaining brain health and preventing cognitive decline.

1. **Reducing Oxidative Stress and Free Radicals**
   Red light therapy has been shown to reduce oxidative stress, a harmful process caused by an excess of free radicals that can damage cells and tissues. This

reduction is crucial for brain health, as oxidative stress is a major contributor to neurodegenerative diseases. By stimulating antioxidant defences and enhancing cellular resilience, RLT may protect the brain against age-related damage and preserve cognitive function.

2. **Protecting Against Neuroinflammation**
Chronic inflammation in the brain is linked to cognitive decline and neurodegenerative diseases. RLT's anti-inflammatory effects can help reduce neuroinflammation, which in turn supports brain health and function. By decreasing inflammation, red light therapy may help prevent or slow the progression of conditions like Alzheimer's and Parkinson's disease, providing a neuroprotective effect that safeguards brain function over time.

3. **Increasing Brain-Derived Neurotrophic Factor (BDNF)**
Brain-derived neurotrophic factor (BDNF) is a protein that promotes the growth,

survival, and differentiation of neurons. BDNF plays a vital role in learning, memory, and higher cognitive functions. Some research suggests that red light therapy may increase BDNF levels, supporting neuronal health and function. Higher BDNF levels help protect against cognitive decline and contribute to mental resilience, enhancing the brain's ability to adapt and recover from stress and injury.

Treating Depression and Mood Disorders with Light Therapy

Light therapy, particularly in the form of red and near-infrared light, has shown promise in managing mood disorders, including depression. It offers a non-invasive approach to treatment that works alongside other therapies or as a standalone tool, depending on the severity of the condition.

1. **Improving Serotonin Levels and Mood**
   Serotonin, often called the "happy hormone," plays a critical role in regulating mood, appetite, and sleep. RLT is thought to enhance serotonin production by stimulating certain neural pathways and increasing blood flow to the brain. Improved serotonin levels are directly linked to a better mood and increased feelings of well-being, making red light therapy a potential tool for those struggling with mood disorders.
2. **Supporting Circadian Rhythms and Sleep-Wake Cycles**
   Many individuals with depression experience disturbances in their circadian rhythms, leading to disrupted sleep patterns and exacerbating symptoms. Red light therapy has been shown to help reset the body's internal clock, improving sleep quality and duration. Better sleep can significantly enhance mood and energy levels, which are often impacted in depressive disorders. By aligning

circadian rhythms, RLT may help those with mood disorders achieve better rest and a more balanced emotional state.

3. **Reducing Symptoms of Seasonal Affective Disorder (SAD)**
Seasonal Affective Disorder (SAD) is a form of depression that typically occurs in the winter months when natural light is limited. Light therapy, including red light therapy, is commonly used to treat SAD by mimicking the natural sunlight needed to regulate mood and energy levels. RLT provides an effective option for individuals with SAD, as it can be administered easily at home and delivers similar benefits to those achieved by full-spectrum light boxes traditionally used for SAD.

4. **Supporting Dopamine and Endorphin Release for Emotional Balance**
RLT may stimulate the release of dopamine and endorphins, neurotransmitters associated with pleasure and well-being. Low levels of these

chemicals are often linked to depressive symptoms, so their enhancement through red light therapy can lead to improved emotional balance and resilience. This neurochemical support allows individuals with mood disorders to experience more stable emotions and an increased ability to manage stress.

Pain Management and Wound Healing with Red Light Therapy

Red light therapy (RLT) is a cutting-edge, non-invasive treatment that has garnered attention for its remarkable effects in pain management and accelerating the healing process of wounds. Through the application of specific wavelengths of red and near-infrared light, RLT promotes cellular regeneration, reduces inflammation, and enhances tissue repair, making it a highly effective therapeutic tool for individuals experiencing chronic pain or recovering from injuries and surgeries.

How Red Light Therapy Alleviates Chronic Pain

Chronic pain can be debilitating, affecting individuals' quality of life and limiting mobility. It is often caused by long-term conditions like arthritis, neuropathy, and muscle strain. Red light therapy offers an innovative approach to managing pain, working at the cellular level to reduce pain perception and enhance healing processes.

1. **Reducing Pain Through Increased Blood Flow**
   One of the primary mechanisms by which red light therapy alleviates pain is by improving blood circulation in the affected area. The light penetrates the skin and tissues, stimulating the production of nitric oxide, a compound that dilates

blood vessels. This dilation increases blood flow to the area, allowing more oxygen and nutrients to reach the damaged tissues, while also helping to remove metabolic waste products that contribute to pain and discomfort. Enhanced circulation promotes a faster recovery process, allowing individuals to experience reduced pain and inflammation.

2. **Modulating Pain Receptors and Nerve Sensitivity**

    Chronic pain often involves heightened sensitivity of the nerves in the affected area. Red light therapy helps modulate the activity of pain receptors in the nervous system, reducing the sensitivity of these nerve endings. By stimulating specific receptors on cells, red light can help desensitise the pain pathways, effectively decreasing the perception of pain. This effect is especially beneficial for those suffering from conditions like neuropathy or fibromyalgia, where nerve pain is a significant symptom.

3. **Triggering Endorphin Production**
Red light therapy may stimulate the production of endorphins, which are natural painkillers produced by the body. Endorphins bind to pain receptors in the brain, reducing the sensation of pain and promoting an overall feeling of well-being. By triggering this natural pain-relief mechanism, red light therapy offers a drug-free way to manage pain without relying on medications that may have unwanted side effects.

Targeting Inflammation for Faster Healing

Inflammation is a key contributor to pain and delayed healing. It is the body's natural response to injury or infection, but chronic or excessive inflammation can impede recovery, cause prolonged discomfort, and even lead to tissue damage. Red light therapy targets the underlying mechanisms of inflammation, reducing it and thereby promoting faster healing.

1. **Reducing Pro-Inflammatory Cytokines**
   Inflammation is regulated by various molecules, including cytokines, which are proteins that signal immune responses and promote inflammation. Red light therapy has been shown to decrease the levels of pro-inflammatory cytokines, which are responsible for the pain, swelling, and redness associated with inflammation. By reducing these cytokines, RLT helps to quell the inflammatory response, allowing tissues to heal more quickly and painlessly.
2. **Enhancing Anti-Inflammatory Pathways**
   In addition to reducing proinflammatory molecules, red light therapy enhances anti-inflammatory pathways. It stimulates the production of certain proteins, such as nuclear factor kappa B (NF-kB), which play a role in suppressing inflammation.

By supporting the body's natural anti-inflammatory processes, RLT can help prevent the escalation of inflammation and enable more efficient tissue recovery.

3. **Reducing Oxidative Stress**
Chronic inflammation is often associated with increased oxidative stress, which occurs when the body produces more free radicals than it can neutralise. Oxidative stress damages healthy cells and tissues, prolonging the healing process. Red light therapy combats oxidative stress by stimulating antioxidant production, neutralising free radicals, and preventing oxidative damage to cells. This reduction in oxidative stress not only alleviates inflammation but also enhances the overall healing process.

Accelerating Recovery from Injuries and Surgeries

Red light therapy is widely used in both clinical and athletic settings to speed up recovery times from injuries and surgeries. Its ability to stimulate cellular repair, reduce inflammation, and enhance tissue regeneration makes it an invaluable tool for post-injury rehabilitation.

1. **Promoting Tissue Regeneration**
   Red light therapy promotes the healing of tissues by stimulating the mitochondria within cells. Mitochondria are responsible for producing energy in the form of ATP, which is essential for cellular repair and regeneration. By increasing ATP production, RLT accelerates the repair of damaged tissues, including muscles, tendons, ligaments, and skin. This is particularly beneficial for individuals recovering from surgical procedures, sports injuries, or trauma, as it speeds up the healing process and reduces the risk of complications.
2. **Reducing Scar Tissue Formation**
   Scar tissue formation is a natural part of

the healing process, but excessive scarring can lead to long-term functional issues or cosmetic concerns. Red light therapy can reduce the formation of excessive scar tissue by promoting the remodelling of collagen and stimulating the growth of healthy tissue. This makes RLT an effective treatment for minimising scarring after surgery or injury, especially in areas like the face, joints, and tendons where scar tissue can impact movement or appearance.

3. **Supporting Bone Healing and Fracture Recovery**
   In cases of bone fractures, red light therapy can stimulate osteoblasts (bone-building cells) and increase the production of collagen, both of which are vital for bone regeneration. By enhancing the healing process at the cellular level, RLT can speed up bone recovery, reducing the time it takes for fractures to heal and decreasing pain associated with bone injuries.

4. **Relieving Post-Surgical Pain and Swelling**

   After surgery, individuals often experience pain and swelling around the incision site, which can delay recovery and cause discomfort. Red light therapy's anti-inflammatory properties help reduce both swelling and pain following surgery, improving the recovery experience. Additionally, by accelerating the repair of tissues and promoting circulation, RLT can help patients regain mobility and function more quickly after surgery.

Success Stories: Using Red Light Therapy for Pain-Free Living

Numerous individuals have experienced life-changing benefits from incorporating red light therapy into their pain management and healing regimens. Here are a few success stories that highlight the potential of RLT in alleviating pain and accelerating recovery:

1. **Chronic Back Pain Relief**
   A patient suffering from chronic lower back pain due to degenerative disc disease found significant relief after incorporating red light therapy into their routine. After several sessions, they reported a marked reduction in pain and stiffness, improved mobility, and an enhanced ability to engage in daily activities without discomfort. The combination of increased circulation and anti-inflammatory effects helped this individual regain a pain-free lifestyle.
2. **Post-Surgery Healing and Scar Reduction**
   A woman who underwent knee surgery for a torn ligament began using red light therapy shortly after her operation. She noticed a reduction in post-surgical swelling, less pain, and faster healing. Within a few months, her knee regained full mobility, and her scar showed minimal signs of scarring. Red light therapy helped accelerate her recovery

and minimise the appearance of the incision.

3. **Sports Injury Recovery for Athletes**
A professional athlete who suffered from chronic tendinitis found red light therapy to be an invaluable tool in her recovery. After a series of RLT sessions, she experienced significant pain relief, improved range of motion, and reduced inflammation in her injured tendon. She was able to return to training faster than expected, and her injury healed with minimal disruption to her performance.

4. **Chronic Shoulder Pain**
A man with chronic shoulder pain due to years of repetitive strain found relief after using red light therapy in conjunction with physical therapy. Over several weeks, the pain in his shoulder decreased significantly, and he regained mobility in the joint. Red light therapy helped reduce the inflammation in the shoulder, facilitating faster healing and less pain during physical activity.

Boosting Immune Function and Overall Health with Red Light Therapy

Red light therapy (RLT) is not only a powerful tool for improving localised pain, skin health, and physical performance but also plays a significant role in strengthening the immune system and enhancing overall well-being. By utilising specific wavelengths of light, RLT can stimulate cellular processes that enhance immune function, reduce inflammation, promote restful sleep, and support hormonal balance.

Strengthening Immunity with Red Light Therapy

The immune system plays a vital role in protecting the body against infections, pathogens, and other harmful agents. A strong immune system is key to maintaining health and preventing diseases, and red light therapy can help support and enhance immune function in several ways:

1. **Stimulating Mitochondria for Energy Production**
   Red light therapy helps stimulate the mitochondria, the energy powerhouses of cells, which play a central role in immune function. Mitochondria produce ATP (adenosine triphosphate), the cellular energy required for immune cells to function efficiently. When mitochondrial

function is optimised through red light exposure, immune cells, such as lymphocytes and macrophages, can respond more quickly and effectively to infections or threats, enhancing the body's immune defence mechanisms.

2. **Increasing Circulation and Lymphatic Drainage**
Improved circulation and lymphatic drainage are critical for a healthy immune response. Red light therapy enhances blood flow by increasing nitric oxide levels, which dilates blood vessels and allows for better oxygen and nutrient delivery to tissues. This improved circulation helps immune cells reach affected areas more quickly, promoting faster responses to infections and inflammation. In addition, red light therapy supports the lymphatic system, which is responsible for removing toxins and waste products from the body, helping to detoxify and strengthen the immune system.

3. **Enhancing White Blood Cell Production**

   Red light therapy has been shown to increase the production of white blood cells (WBCs), which are key players in the immune response. WBCs are responsible for identifying and attacking pathogens, viruses, and other harmful invaders. By stimulating the production of these immune cells, RLT can help the body mount a more effective defence against infections and illnesses.

4. **Boosting Antioxidant Defences**

   Red light therapy also supports the production of antioxidants in the body, which are essential for neutralising harmful free radicals. Free radicals can damage cells and weaken the immune system, leading to chronic inflammation and disease. By enhancing the body's natural antioxidant defences, red light therapy helps protect immune cells from oxidative stress, ensuring they remain effective in responding to threats.

Reducing Inflammatory Markers and Disease Prevention

Inflammation is a natural response to injury or infection, but when it becomes chronic or excessive, it can contribute to various health problems, including autoimmune diseases, cardiovascular conditions, and cancer. Reducing inflammation is crucial for preventing disease and promoting long-term health. Red light therapy plays a key role in regulating inflammatory markers and reducing chronic inflammation throughout the body.

1. **Modulating Inflammatory Pathways**
   Chronic inflammation is often caused by an overactive immune system that continually releases inflammatory molecules such as cytokines and prostaglandins. Red light therapy helps modulate these inflammatory pathways by influencing key signalling molecules that control inflammation. Studies have shown

that RLT can reduce the production of pro-inflammatory cytokines, which are responsible for inflammation and the symptoms of various inflammatory conditions, including arthritis, asthma, and chronic pain.
2. **Reducing C-Reactive Protein (CRP)**
C-reactive protein (CRP) is a common biomarker for inflammation in the body. High CRP levels are associated with an increased risk of cardiovascular disease, diabetes, and other chronic conditions. Red light therapy has been shown to reduce CRP levels, indicating a reduction in systemic inflammation. By lowering CRP, RLT helps to reduce the overall inflammatory load on the body, which can help prevent the development of chronic diseases linked to inflammation.
3. **Supporting Immune System Homeostasis**
Red light therapy helps maintain immune system homeostasis, ensuring that the immune system is neither overactive nor

underactive. By stimulating the production of anti-inflammatory molecules and enhancing cellular function, RLT supports the immune system in managing its responses to pathogens and threats. This balanced immune response can help prevent chronic inflammatory diseases and promote better overall health.

Promoting Better Sleep and Recovery Cycles

Sleep is one of the most important factors for maintaining optimal health. During sleep, the body undergoes critical repair processes, including tissue regeneration, immune system strengthening, and memory consolidation. Red light therapy has been shown to support better sleep quality, enhance recovery cycles, and promote restful, rejuvenating sleep.

1. **Regulating Circadian Rhythms and Melatonin Production**

Exposure to red and near-infrared light can help regulate the body's circadian rhythms, which govern the sleep-wake cycle. Red light therapy stimulates the production of melatonin, a hormone that is essential for sleep. Unlike blue light, which can suppress melatonin production and interfere with sleep, red light does not disrupt melatonin secretion and can even promote its production. By supporting melatonin levels, RLT can help individuals fall asleep faster, stay asleep longer, and enjoy deeper, more restorative sleep.

2. **Improving Sleep Quality and Duration**
   Studies have shown that red light therapy can improve sleep quality by increasing the amount of time spent in the deep sleep stages, such as REM sleep. Deep sleep is when the body performs essential restorative processes, including muscle repair, immune strengthening, and tissue regeneration. By enhancing the deep sleep cycle, RLT promotes faster recovery and

rejuvenation, allowing the body to repair itself more effectively.

3. **Reducing Sleep Disruptions in Chronic Pain Conditions**
For individuals suffering from chronic pain, sleep disturbances are a common issue. Pain can prevent individuals from falling asleep or staying asleep, leading to fatigue and slower recovery. Red light therapy, with its pain-relieving and anti-inflammatory properties, helps reduce the intensity of chronic pain, making it easier for individuals to sleep soundly and wake up feeling refreshed and restored.

Supporting Hormonal Balance and Metabolic Health

Hormonal imbalances and metabolic disorders can have far-reaching effects on overall health, influencing mood, energy levels, body composition, and the risk of chronic conditions. Red light therapy plays a crucial role in supporting hormonal balance and metabolic health by influencing various physiological processes at the cellular level.

1. **Supporting Thyroid Health and Function**
   The thyroid gland plays a key role in regulating metabolism, energy production, and hormonal balance. Red light therapy has been shown to help support thyroid function by improving mitochondrial activity and reducing oxidative stress. By promoting efficient energy production in thyroid cells, RLT can help improve metabolic function and prevent issues related to thyroid dysfunction, such as hypothyroidism or hyperthyroidism.
2. **Balancing Cortisol Levels**
   Cortisol, often referred to as the "stress hormone," is produced by the adrenal glands in response to stress. While cortisol is essential for managing short-term stress, chronic high cortisol levels can disrupt sleep, promote weight gain, and impair

immune function. Red light therapy has been shown to help regulate cortisol production, reducing the negative effects of chronic stress and promoting a healthier hormonal balance.

3. **Promoting Insulin Sensitivity**
Insulin resistance is a major risk factor for the development of type 2 diabetes and other metabolic disorders. Red light therapy has been found to enhance insulin sensitivity by improving cellular function and glucose uptake. This can help reduce the risk of diabetes and support healthy metabolism, making it an important tool for managing blood sugar levels and maintaining a healthy weight.

4. **Supporting Female Hormones**
Red light therapy has also been shown to benefit women by supporting hormonal balance during menopause or other hormonal fluctuations. By enhancing circulation, reducing stress, and supporting endocrine function, RLT can help alleviate symptoms of hormonal

Healing With Red Light Therapy

imbalances, such as hot flashes, fatigue, and mood swings.

Sexual Health and Fertility Enhancement with Red Light Therapy

Red light therapy (RLT) has increasingly become a valuable tool in enhancing sexual health and supporting fertility. By utilising specific wavelengths of red and near-infrared light, RLT can stimulate a variety of physiological processes in the body that promote reproductive health, improve libido, and optimise overall sexual function.

Benefits for Reproductive Health and Libido

Sexual health encompasses a range of factors, including hormonal balance, sexual function, libido, and reproductive capacity. Many individuals experience issues in these areas due to ageing, stress, lifestyle factors, or underlying health conditions. Red light therapy offers numerous benefits for improving sexual health, particularly in terms of libido, reproductive health, and overall sexual vitality.

1. **Enhancing Hormonal Balance**
   One of the key mechanisms through which red light therapy supports sexual health is by helping regulate hormonal balance. Hormones like testosterone, oestrogen, and progesterone play critical roles in regulating sexual desire, function, and overall reproductive health. Red light therapy stimulates mitochondrial function in hormone-producing glands, such as the ovaries and testes, enhancing their ability

to produce key hormones. This can lead to improvements in libido and sexual performance, particularly in individuals experiencing low sexual desire due to hormonal imbalances or ageing.

2. **Boosting Testosterone Levels**
   Testosterone is a critical hormone for both male and female sexual health. In men, it plays a central role in libido, erectile function, and overall sexual vitality. In women, testosterone contributes to sexual desire and overall energy levels. Red light therapy has been shown to increase testosterone production by stimulating the Leydig cells in the testes in men and the ovaries in women. This increase in testosterone can lead to a natural enhancement of libido, energy, and overall sexual well-being.

3. **Increasing Libido and Sexual Desire**
   Libido can be affected by a variety of factors, including stress, fatigue, ageing, and hormonal imbalances. Red light therapy has been found to improve

circulation and reduce stress, two key factors that contribute to a healthy libido. By increasing blood flow to the pelvic region and supporting hormonal balance, RLT can help individuals feel more sexually confident, spontaneous, and connected to their partners.

Using Red Light Therapy to Support Fertility

Fertility challenges affect millions of people around the world, with factors like stress, age, lifestyle, and health conditions playing a role in both male and female fertility. Red light therapy has emerged as a promising non-invasive treatment option for improving fertility by addressing several key physiological factors that influence reproductive health.

1. **Improving Ovarian Function and Egg Quality (Women)**
   For women, red light therapy has been shown to support ovarian function,

including improving the quality and quantity of eggs. By stimulating mitochondrial activity, RLT enhances the energy production necessary for optimal cellular function. This effect extends to the reproductive cells, supporting the health of eggs and improving the chances of successful conception. In studies, women undergoing red light therapy have reported improved menstrual cycles, more consistent ovulation, and better outcomes in assisted reproductive technologies like in vitro fertilisation (IVF).

2. **Supporting Sperm Health and Count (Men)**
Male fertility is often linked to sperm health, including sperm count, motility, and morphology. Red light therapy has demonstrated promising effects in improving these factors by increasing circulation to the testes and stimulating mitochondrial function in sperm cells. By optimising mitochondrial activity, RLT helps improve sperm energy production,

which is essential for motility and overall sperm quality. In several studies, men undergoing RLT have reported improvements in sperm count and motility, contributing to a higher chance of successful conception.

3. **Improving Blood Flow to the Reproductive Organs**
Healthy blood flow to the reproductive organs is essential for both male and female fertility. Red light therapy increases blood circulation by enhancing nitric oxide production, which dilates blood vessels and improves oxygen and nutrient delivery to tissues. This improved circulation supports the reproductive organs, ensuring they receive the necessary nutrients and oxygen to function optimally. This is particularly important for individuals with conditions such as erectile dysfunction or poor ovarian blood flow, both of which can hinder fertility.

4. **Reducing Inflammation for Better Reproductive Health**

   Inflammation is often a significant barrier to fertility. Conditions such as endometriosis, polycystic ovary syndrome (PCOS), and male infertility can all be exacerbated by chronic inflammation. Red light therapy has potent anti-inflammatory effects, helping to reduce systemic inflammation and promote healthier reproductive organs. By regulating the inflammatory response, RLT can improve conditions related to infertility, contributing to better fertility outcomes.

Improving Circulation and Blood Flow for Sexual Function

Optimal sexual function relies heavily on adequate blood flow to the genital area, as well as the ability of the cardiovascular system to respond to arousal signals. Red light therapy's ability to enhance circulation is a major factor in improving sexual performance, particularly for individuals experiencing erectile dysfunction (ED) or poor sexual arousal due to circulation issues.

1. **Red Light for Erectile Dysfunction (ED)**
   Erectile dysfunction is a common issue for men, often caused by poor blood flow to the penis. Red light therapy helps improve circulation by stimulating nitric oxide production, which dilates blood vessels and enhances blood flow. This can result in stronger, longer-lasting erections and improved erectile function. Studies have shown that men with ED who underwent red light therapy experienced significant improvements in erectile function, suggesting that RLT can be an effective alternative or complement to traditional ED treatments.
2. **Enhancing Female Sexual Arousal**
   For women, sexual arousal is strongly influenced by blood flow to the genital area. Poor circulation can result in

decreased arousal, vaginal dryness, and difficulty reaching orgasm. Red light therapy increases blood flow to the vaginal and pelvic region, which may help with vaginal lubrication and overall sexual enjoyment. Additionally, by improving blood flow and reducing inflammation, RLT can contribute to a more pleasurable and satisfying sexual experience for women.

3. **Boosting Sensitivity and Sexual Pleasure**

    Increased blood flow to the sexual organs not only enhances physical arousal but also increases sensitivity, making sexual experiences more enjoyable. Red light therapy's ability to stimulate circulation can improve nerve function and increase sensitivity in the genital area, leading to more intense pleasure during intimate moments. This is particularly beneficial for individuals who may experience diminished sensation due to age, hormonal imbalances, or health conditions.

Real-Life Accounts of Red Light Therapy's Impact on Intimacy

While scientific studies provide evidence of the benefits of red light therapy, personal success stories are often the most convincing testament to its effectiveness in real-world scenarios. Below are a few realistic and believable accounts of individuals who have experienced significant improvements in sexual health and intimacy as a result of using red light therapy.

1. **Case Study 1: Sarah and Tim's Journey to Improved Fertility**
   Sarah, 32, and her partner Tim, 34, had been trying to conceive for over a year without success. After consulting with a fertility specialist, they decided to incorporate red light therapy into their routine to improve Sarah's egg quality and Tim's sperm count. Within three months of using red light therapy, Sarah noticed her menstrual cycles became more regular,

and she experienced less cramping. Tim reported an increase in his sperm motility, which was confirmed through semen analysis. After six months, Sarah conceived naturally, a result they attribute in part to the benefits of red light therapy in supporting their reproductive health.

2. **Case Study 2: Mark's Experience with Erectile Dysfunction**
Mark, 48, had been dealing with erectile dysfunction for several years, primarily caused by poor circulation and stress. Despite trying medications and lifestyle changes, he found little improvement. After learning about red light therapy, he decided to try it as a natural, non-invasive option. After three weeks of using a red light therapy device for just 10 minutes daily, Mark noticed significant improvements in his ability to achieve and maintain an erection. He also reported feeling more confident in his sexual performance and enjoyed more satisfying intimate experiences with his partner.

Mark continues to use red light therapy regularly as part of his overall sexual health routine.

3. **Case Study 3: Maria's Renewed Libido and Intimacy**

   Maria, 39, had noticed a significant decline in her libido after experiencing stress at work and during menopause. She felt disconnected from her partner and began to lose interest in intimacy. After incorporating red light therapy into her daily routine, Maria experienced a noticeable improvement in her libido. She also reported feeling more energised and less stressed, which helped rekindle the intimacy in her relationship. Maria's partner also noted a difference in their sexual connection, and they both experienced a more fulfilling and passionate relationship as a result of the positive effects of red light therapy.

Setting Up Red Light Therapy at Home

Red light therapy (RLT) is a powerful tool for improving a wide range of health concerns, from skin rejuvenation to pain management, muscle recovery, and even improving mental health. One of the most appealing aspects of red light therapy is the convenience of using it at home. Setting up a home RLT system can be straightforward if you know what to look for and follow some key guidelines.

Choosing the Right Red Light Therapy Device

The first step in setting up red light therapy at home is selecting the right device. There are many options available on the market, ranging from handheld devices to large panels or full-body units. The type of device you choose will depend on your specific needs, budget, and the area of your body you wish to treat. Here are a few factors to consider:

1. **Device Type**
    - **Handheld Devices**: These are small, portable units that are ideal for localised treatments, such as targeting small areas like the face, joints, or specific muscle groups. Handheld devices are often more affordable but may require longer sessions to cover a broader area.
    - **Panel or Lamp Devices**: These are larger units that cover a broader area at once. They are ideal for treating larger sections of the body, like the back or legs. Many panel

devices come with adjustable stands for easier positioning.
- **Full-Body Systems**: For individuals looking for a more comprehensive, full-body treatment, there are full-body red light therapy systems. These are more expensive but offer the advantage of treating the entire body simultaneously. They are often used in professional clinics and gyms but can also be installed at home.

2. **Wavelength and Spectrum**

The most effective wavelengths for red light therapy fall between 600 and 1,000 nanometers (nm). Here's what you need to know about choosing the right wavelength:
- **Red Light (600-650 nm)**: Red light is best for surface-level treatments, such as improving skin health, reducing wrinkles, and enhancing collagen production. It's also

beneficial for reducing superficial pain and inflammation.
- **Near-Infrared Light (800-850 nm)**: This wavelength penetrates deeper into the tissues and is ideal for treating deeper muscles, joints, and bones. Near-infrared light is particularly effective for healing injuries, reducing inflammation, and accelerating muscle recovery.

3. **Important Note**: Many devices offer a combination of red and near-infrared light, which can be advantageous depending on the condition being treated. Ensure that the device you choose provides the right wavelength for your intended use.
4. **Power Output and Intensity**

The power output of the device is measured in milliwatts per square centimetre (mW/cm^2). The higher the power output, the more intense the light, which generally means a shorter treatment time is required. However, higher power

output can also increase the risk of skin damage if used improperly.
- **Low Power**: Ideal for skin rejuvenation, hair regrowth, and mild pain relief. These devices generally require longer exposure times.
- **High Power**: Suitable for deeper tissue treatment and faster results, especially for conditions like joint pain, muscle recovery, and inflammation. Higher-powered devices are more commonly found in clinical settings but are available for home use as well.

5. **Size and Coverage Area**

   If you plan to treat large areas, such as your back or legs, a larger panel will be necessary to cover more space at once. Smaller handheld devices are good for spot treatments but might not be ideal for larger areas.

6. **Price and Durability**

   Red light therapy devices vary in price,

with handheld devices starting at around $50 and full-body panels costing over $1,000. While it's important to stick to your budget, be sure to prioritise quality. Look for devices with durable construction, proper certifications (such as FDA-cleared), and reliable customer support.

Understanding Light Wavelengths and Intensity Levels

When setting up red light therapy at home, understanding the specific wavelengths and intensity levels is crucial to maximising its effectiveness. As mentioned earlier, red and near-infrared wavelengths are the most commonly used for therapeutic purposes.

- **Red Light (600-650 nm)**: This wavelength targets superficial skin layers and is effective for promoting skin health, reducing fine lines, wrinkles, and redness,

and enhancing collagen production. It also helps with minor pain relief and can accelerate wound healing.
- **Near-Infrared Light (800-850 nm)**: This wavelength penetrates deeper into muscles, joints, and bones, providing healing for deeper tissues, reducing inflammation, and supporting muscle recovery. It is often used for conditions like arthritis, muscle strains, and joint pain.

Intensity: Red light therapy devices can vary in intensity, which directly impacts the effectiveness of the treatment. Devices with higher intensity can provide faster results, but they also carry a higher risk of skin damage if misused. Lower intensity devices may require longer exposure times to achieve the desired effects.

- **Moderate Intensity (30-100 mW/cm^2)**: This is generally sufficient for most skin rejuvenation, hair growth, and pain relief treatments.

- **High Intensity (100-200 mW/cm²)**: Ideal for muscle recovery, joint pain, and deeper tissue treatments.

Always refer to the device's user manual for guidelines on intensity settings, and ensure you follow the recommended duration for each session.

Placement, Positioning, and Setup Tips

Proper placement and positioning of your red light therapy device are essential for ensuring you get the most out of your treatments. Incorrect positioning can lead to uneven exposure, reduced effectiveness, and even safety risks.

1. **Distance from the Body**
   The optimal distance between the device and the body depends on the device's power output. For most handheld devices, the recommended distance is 6-12 inches, while panel devices may need to be

positioned a bit further away—typically 12-24 inches. Be sure to follow the manufacturer's guidelines for the correct distance.

2. **Treatment Area**
    - **For Localised Treatment**: Hold the device or position it to target specific areas, such as a joint, muscle, or your face. If you're treating a specific injury, you may want to concentrate the light directly on the area for maximum effect.
    - **For Full-Body Treatment**: If you're using a full-body panel, ensure the light is positioned to cover as much of your body as possible. For optimal results, keep the device stationary at a height that allows the light to shine directly onto the target areas. Some full-body panels come with adjustable stands for easy positioning.

3. **Treatment Duration**

   Treatment times vary depending on the type of device and the area being treated. For most devices, a session may last anywhere from 5 to 20 minutes. Start with shorter sessions and gradually increase the duration to avoid overstimulation. A typical regimen is 3-5 times per week for optimal results.

4. **Consistency is Key**

   Just like with any therapy, consistency is crucial. Results from red light therapy are not instant and may take several weeks of consistent use to notice significant improvements. Create a schedule that works for you and stick to it.

Avoiding Common Mistakes: Safety Tips and Precautions

While red light therapy is generally safe, it's important to follow certain safety guidelines to avoid injury or ineffective treatment. Below are some tips to ensure that you use your device properly and safely.

1. **Avoid Overexposure**
   Overexposure to red light therapy can lead to skin irritation or burns, particularly if the device is too powerful or used for too long. Stick to the recommended treatment duration and intensity.
2. **Use Protective Eyewear**
   Although red and near-infrared light is non-invasive, the intensity can still cause eye strain or damage if exposed for long periods. Wear protective goggles to safeguard your eyes, especially when using high-intensity devices or when targeting the face. Many devices come with goggles or recommend specific eye protection.
3. **Don't Use on Injured Skin**
   Avoid using red light therapy on open wounds, irritated skin, or sunburned areas. RLT can promote healing, but it should be used with caution on sensitive or injured

skin. Always wait for skin to heal before resuming treatments.

4. **Consult with a Healthcare Professional**
   If you have any underlying health conditions, such as cancer, photosensitivity, or skin disorders, consult with your healthcare provider before starting red light therapy. People who are pregnant or have epilepsy should also avoid using certain wavelengths without medical advice.

5. **Monitor Progress**
   Track your progress to see how your body responds to red light therapy. If you experience any discomfort, pain, or adverse reactions, reduce the intensity or duration of your sessions or consult a healthcare provider.

How to Use Red Light Therapy Effectively

Red light therapy (RLT) has been shown to offer a variety of health benefits, ranging from pain relief and enhanced muscle recovery to improving skin health and mental clarity. However, to maximise the therapeutic effects of this powerful tool, it is essential to use it effectively. This involves understanding the optimal timing, distance, and duration of treatments, as well as creating customised protocols to address specific health concerns.

Step-by-Step Guide to Treatment Timing and Frequency

To achieve the most effective results from red light therapy, it is important to follow a consistent treatment schedule. The frequency and timing of your sessions will depend on the condition you're addressing, the device you're using, and your body's response to the therapy. Below is a general guide to treatment timing and frequency:

1. **Frequency of Sessions**
   - **General Skin Rejuvenation**: For skin-related concerns such as wrinkles, acne, or scars, it's recommended to use red light therapy 3-5 times per week for about 10-20 minutes per session. The skin can regenerate quickly, so consistent use is key to seeing improvements over time.
   - **Pain Relief and Muscle Recovery**: If you're using red light therapy for pain management, joint pain, or

muscle recovery, the ideal frequency is 3-4 times per week. For more severe or chronic conditions, you may want to start with daily sessions and reduce the frequency once improvements are noticed.
- **Deep Tissue and Injury Recovery**: When treating deeper injuries, such as ligament sprains or deep muscle tears, it is often beneficial to start with a higher frequency (daily or every other day) to speed up the healing process. Once the condition improves, you can reduce the frequency to 2-3 times per week.
- **Mental Health and Cognitive Enhancement**: For issues like anxiety, depression, or mental clarity, use red light therapy 3-5 times per week, with each session lasting around 10-15 minutes. This helps stimulate brain activity and promotes neurogenesis.

2. **Timing of Sessions**
    - Red light therapy can be done at any time of the day; however, certain times may be more beneficial depending on the issue you're addressing. For example, if you're using RLT to improve sleep quality or reduce stress, it may be best to schedule your sessions in the evening or before bed.
    - For pain relief or muscle recovery, RLT can be done before or after workouts, depending on your specific needs. Many people prefer to use it post-workout to help reduce soreness and inflammation.
3. **Consistency** Red light therapy works by stimulating the body's healing mechanisms, which takes time. Just as with any therapeutic treatment, consistency is essential for seeing long-term results. It's important to commit to a regular schedule and stick with it for

several weeks before reassessing your progress.

Optimal Distance and Duration for Different Conditions

The optimal distance from the device and the duration of each treatment session can vary depending on the condition you're targeting and the type of device you're using. Here are some general guidelines for different uses of red light therapy:

1. **For Skin Health (Acne, Wrinkles, and Collagen Production)**
   - **Distance**: 6-12 inches (15-30 cm) from the device.
   - **Duration**: 10-20 minutes per session.
   - **Frequency**: 3-5 times per week.
2. **Tip**: For acne treatment, it may be helpful to focus on problem areas, using a handheld device to target the face or

specific blemishes. For wrinkle reduction or overall skin rejuvenation, try using a panel device to cover a larger area of the face or body.
3. **For Muscle Recovery and Performance**
    - **Distance**: 12-18 inches (30-45 cm) from the device.
    - **Duration**: 10-20 minutes for a localised area or 20-30 minutes for a larger area.
    - **Frequency**: Daily or 3-4 times per week, depending on the severity of the condition.
4. **Tip**: After workouts or physical activity, use red light therapy to focus on muscle groups that are sore or have been worked the hardest. You can also use red light therapy before exercise to increase blood circulation and reduce the risk of injury.
5. **For Joint and Pain Relief (Arthritis, Injuries, Inflammation)**
    - **Distance**: 12-24 inches (30-60 cm), depending on the size of the joint or area being treated.

- **Duration**: 10-15 minutes per treatment area.
     - **Frequency**: 3-4 times per week or daily for chronic pain.
6. **Tip**: Position the device directly over the painful area, ensuring the light is penetrating the joint or muscle deeply. If you are treating a large area, ensure that the light covers the entire affected area.
7. **For Mental Clarity and Brain Health**
     - **Distance**: 6-12 inches (15-30 cm) from the device if using a handheld or smaller unit.
     - **Duration**: 10-15 minutes per session.
     - **Frequency**: 3-5 times per week.
8. **Tip**: Red light therapy for brain health often involves shining the light on the head, particularly the forehead or temples. Sessions can be done before bed to promote relaxation and mental clarity or in the morning for an energy boost.

Customised Protocols for Pain, Skin, Fitness, and More

While red light therapy can be used for a wide range of health benefits, customising your protocol based on your specific needs is crucial to achieve optimal results. Below are some examples of how you can tailor your red light therapy regimen for different goals:

1. **Pain and Inflammation Protocol**
    - **Goal**: Alleviate chronic pain and reduce inflammation.
    - **Device Type**: Large panel device or handheld for localised treatment.
    - **Protocol**:
        - Use 10-15 minutes per treatment area.
        - Focus on the area of pain, such as knees, back, or shoulders.
        - Apply 3-4 times per week or daily for severe pain.
    - **Tip**: For deeper tissue pain, consider using near-infrared light,

which penetrates deeper into the muscles and joints.
2. **Skin Rejuvenation Protocol**
    - **Goal**: Improve skin tone, texture, and reduce wrinkles.
    - **Device Type**: Panel device for large surface areas or handheld for smaller areas.
    - **Protocol**:
        - Use 10-20 minutes for each treatment area (face, neck, chest).
        - Focus on areas with wrinkles or pigmentation.
        - Apply 3-5 times per week.
    - **Tip**: For acne, consider adding blue light therapy, which has been shown to be effective in killing acne-causing bacteria.
3. **Fitness and Muscle Recovery Protocol**
    - **Goal**: Speed up muscle recovery and enhance performance.
    - **Device Type**: Full-body panel or handheld device.

- Protocol:
    - Use 15-20 minutes on each targeted muscle group after workouts.
    - Focus on areas with muscle soreness or stiffness.
    - Apply 3-4 times per week.
- Tip: Use RLT for pre-workout sessions to improve circulation and post-workout to reduce soreness and inflammation.

4. **Mental Clarity and Brain Health Protocol**
    - **Goal**: Enhance memory, focus, and reduce mental fatigue.
    - **Device Type**: Handheld device or small panel.
    - **Protocol**:
        - Use 10-15 minutes focusing on the head area (forehead or temples).
        - Apply 3-5 times per week, preferably in the morning or

before a mentally demanding task.
- **Tip**: Combine RLT with deep breathing or meditation to maximise relaxation and cognitive benefits.

Tracking Your Progress and Adjusting Your Routine

Tracking your progress is essential to determine whether red light therapy is working for you and to adjust your routine as needed. Here are some strategies for monitoring your results:

1. **Keep a Journal**
   - Record your sessions: Note the duration, intensity, and area treated for each session.
   - Track any changes in symptoms: For example, if you're treating pain, note if there's any reduction in

discomfort or improved range of motion.
2. **Monitor Skin Changes**
    - Take "before" and "after" photos to track improvements in skin tone, wrinkles, or acne.
    - Look for gradual changes over a few weeks—results with skin care treatments often take time.
3. **Adjust Based on Results**
    - If you aren't seeing the desired effects, adjust the frequency, duration, or intensity.
    - Increase the frequency if you need faster results or decrease it if you feel your body needs more recovery time.
4. **Consult with a Professional**
    - If you experience any adverse reactions or if your progress plateaus, consult a healthcare professional who can help you tweak your protocol for better results.

Maximising Results with Red Light Therapy

Red light therapy (RLT) is a powerful and versatile treatment that can enhance many aspects of health and wellness, including skin rejuvenation, pain relief, muscle recovery, mental clarity, and more. However, to achieve the maximum benefits from this therapy, it's essential to integrate it with other health practices. Combining red light therapy with proper nutrition, exercise, complementary therapies, and lifestyle adjustments can significantly accelerate results and improve overall well-being.

Combining Red Light Therapy with Nutrition and Supplements

While red light therapy works by stimulating cellular energy production and promoting healing, its effects can be enhanced when combined with the right nutrition and supplements. The body needs proper fuel to repair and regenerate tissues, reduce inflammation, and support overall function. Here's how you can optimise your results with a nutrient-rich diet and targeted supplements:

1. **Nutrition for Skin Health and Anti-Aging**
    - **Collagen-Boosting Foods**: Collagen is a key structural protein in the skin, and red light therapy promotes collagen production. To further enhance skin rejuvenation, include collagen-rich foods like bone broth, fish, chicken skin, and eggs in your diet. You can also take

collagen supplements to help your body produce more of this vital protein.
- **Vitamin C**: As an antioxidant, vitamin C plays a crucial role in collagen synthesis and helps fight free radicals that cause skin ageing. Incorporate foods like citrus fruits, strawberries, bell peppers, and broccoli to ensure sufficient vitamin C intake.
- **Healthy Fats**: Omega-3 fatty acids, found in fatty fish (such as salmon), flaxseeds, and walnuts, reduce inflammation and promote healthy skin. Healthy fats also support the cellular membranes, helping red light penetrate cells more effectively.
- **Antioxidant-Rich Foods**: Red light therapy stimulates healing and cell regeneration, which can be enhanced by antioxidants. Blueberries, spinach, kale, and dark

chocolate are rich in antioxidants that fight oxidative stress and protect cells from damage.
2. **Supplements to Enhance Red Light Therapy Effects**
    - **Vitamin D**: Red light therapy can help regulate the immune system, and vitamin D is a key factor in immune function. Supplementing with vitamin D, especially if you live in areas with limited sunlight, can improve overall immune health.
    - **Magnesium**: Known for its muscle-relaxing properties, magnesium helps reduce muscle soreness and enhances the effectiveness of red light therapy for muscle recovery. Magnesium also promotes better sleep, which supports overall healing.
    - **CoQ10 (Coenzyme Q10)**: CoQ10 is involved in cellular energy production, and its supplementation can complement the

energy-boosting effects of red light therapy. It is particularly beneficial for ageing individuals, as CoQ10 levels naturally decrease with age.
- **Turmeric and Curcumin**: These natural anti-inflammatory compounds can help reduce pain and inflammation, enhancing red light therapy's effectiveness for pain management and recovery.

By fueling your body with these essential nutrients and supplements, you can help optimise your body's healing processes and maximise the benefits of red light therapy.

Complementary Therapies: Exercise, Meditation, and More

Integrating red light therapy with other health-promoting practices can create a synergistic effect, enhancing the results you achieve. Combining RLT with exercise, meditation, and other complementary therapies can accelerate recovery, reduce stress, and improve mental clarity.

1. **Exercise and Red Light Therapy**
   - **Pre-Workout Activation**: Red light therapy can be used before exercise to improve circulation, enhance energy production at the cellular level, and prepare muscles for the physical demands ahead. For example, using RLT for 10-15 minutes before a workout may increase endurance, reduce muscle fatigue, and promote better performance during your workout.
   - **Post-Workout Recovery**: After exercise, red light therapy helps reduce inflammation, muscle soreness, and accelerates recovery by increasing circulation and oxygen delivery to tissues. For best results, use red light therapy immediately after your workout for

15-20 minutes on the muscle groups that were targeted during exercise.
- **Consistency**: Regular physical activity combined with red light therapy helps maintain long-term muscle health, reduce the risk of injury, and prevent the loss of strength over time.

2. **Meditation and Mindfulness with Red Light Therapy**
   - **Stress Reduction**: Meditation and mindfulness practices can significantly reduce stress and anxiety, improving overall well-being. When combined with red light therapy, which can also help reduce stress and promote relaxation, the two therapies complement each other. Consider using RLT as part of your meditation routine to enhance relaxation and calm the mind.
   - **Boosting Brain Health**: Red light therapy is beneficial for cognitive

function, but pairing it with mindfulness practices can further promote mental clarity, focus, and concentration. Meditation can help you stay centred and calm while RLT stimulates brain activity and neurogenesis.
  - **Better Sleep**: Meditation practices before or after using red light therapy can support deeper sleep and help reset your circadian rhythm. Both therapies contribute to reduced stress levels, making it easier to unwind and improve sleep quality.
3. **Other Complementary Therapies**
   - **Massage Therapy**: Incorporating massage therapy with red light therapy enhances tissue relaxation, accelerates muscle recovery, and promotes blood circulation. RLT can help speed up the healing of muscles and joints after a deep tissue massage, and the

combination of both therapies can reduce pain and stiffness.
- **Cryotherapy**: Cold therapy (cryotherapy) is often used after intense physical activity to reduce inflammation and accelerate muscle recovery. When used in conjunction with red light therapy, cryotherapy helps further reduce pain and inflammation while RLT works to promote tissue repair and regeneration.

By integrating these complementary therapies with red light therapy, you create a well-rounded approach to improving your health, reducing stress, and enhancing your physical and mental well-being.

Enhancing Results Through Lifestyle Adjustments

Healing With Red Light Therapy

In addition to combining red light therapy with nutrition, exercise, and other therapies, making lifestyle adjustments can further enhance the effectiveness of your RLT sessions. Here are some lifestyle habits that can complement your therapy and boost results:

1. **Get Enough Sleep**
    - Sleep is when your body does most of its repair and recovery. Red light therapy stimulates cellular regeneration, and getting adequate rest supports that process. Aim for 7-9 hours of sleep each night to allow your body to fully recover and benefit from the therapeutic effects of RLT.
2. **Hydrate Well**
    - Red light therapy stimulates cellular activity, which requires water. Staying well-hydrated ensures that cells can function optimally, allowing nutrients to be absorbed and toxins to be flushed out.

Drinking plenty of water before and after your RLT sessions can help improve the effectiveness of the therapy.

3. **Reduce Stress**
   - Chronic stress has a negative impact on health, impeding the body's ability to heal and recover. Use relaxation techniques such as deep breathing, yoga, and mindfulness to manage stress levels. The less stressed you are, the more effective red light therapy will be in promoting healing and well-being.

4. **Minimise Exposure to Toxins**
   - Exposure to environmental toxins, such as air pollution, chemicals, and processed foods, can interfere with your body's healing process. Reducing exposure to harmful substances can help your body repair and regenerate more

effectively, making red light therapy work even better.

Tools for Monitoring Health Improvements

To track your progress and ensure that you're getting the most out of your red light therapy sessions, it's helpful to use tools that can monitor various health metrics. Here are some tools to help you monitor your improvements:

1. **Skin Health Tracking Apps**
    - Use smartphone apps to track changes in your skin, such as reductions in wrinkles, acne, and pigmentation. Some apps allow you to take photos over time and compare them to monitor visible improvements.
2. **Pain and Recovery Journals**
    - For pain management and muscle recovery, keeping a journal can be an effective way to track your

symptoms. Write down your pain levels before and after each red light therapy session, along with any changes in inflammation, soreness, or muscle stiffness.

3. **Wearable Fitness Devices**
    - Wearables like fitness trackers and smartwatches can track heart rate, sleep patterns, steps, and overall activity levels. Monitoring these metrics can help you assess how red light therapy affects your physical performance, recovery, and general well-being.
4. **Mood and Cognitive Function Trackers**
    - Apps that track mood, mental clarity, or cognitive function can be helpful for monitoring the effects of red light therapy on mental health. Tracking your mood over time will allow you to see improvements in stress, anxiety, and overall brain function as you integrate red light therapy into your routine.

Exploring Advanced Red Light Therapy Techniques

While traditional red light therapy (RLT) is highly effective for a range of common health conditions, the therapy's true potential is often realised when combined with advanced techniques and complementary treatments. Exploring advanced red light therapy techniques not only expands the possibilities for its application but also enhances the overall effectiveness of treatments for complex health conditions. In this section, we will look into various advanced methods, including using red light therapy in conjunction with near-infrared light, combining it with other therapeutic modalities like cold therapy and saunas, and examining its potential for addressing more complex health challenges. We will also touch on emerging trends and experimental applications of red light therapy in cutting-edge medical research.

Using Red Light Therapy in Conjunction with Near-Infrared Light

One of the most advanced techniques in red light therapy involves the use of **near-infrared (NIR) light** alongside traditional red light wavelengths. Near-infrared light typically falls in the range of 700–1,100 nanometers, while red light is usually in the range of 600–700 nanometers. When combined, the two types of light can provide enhanced benefits for deeper tissues and offer a broader spectrum of healing.

1. **Why Combine Red and Near-Infrared Light?**
    - **Penetration Depth**: Red light is more effective at targeting superficial tissues like the skin, while near-infrared light can penetrate deeper into muscles, joints, and even bones. Using both types of light allows for comprehensive treatment that addresses both surface-level and deeper health concerns simultaneously.
    - **Synergistic Effects**: The combination of red and near-infrared light can stimulate a broader range of cellular responses. Red light therapy promotes collagen production and reduces inflammation at the surface level, while near-infrared light targets deeper tissues to accelerate healing, reduce muscle soreness, and improve joint function.

- **Enhanced Cellular Energy**: Near-infrared light specifically stimulates the **mitochondria**, which are responsible for producing energy (ATP) in cells. When combined with red light therapy, it boosts cellular energy and facilitates faster tissue regeneration and recovery.

2. **Application in Treatment**
   - **Pain and Inflammation**: Combining red and near-infrared light is particularly useful for conditions involving deep pain, such as muscle strains, joint pain, arthritis, and tendonitis. The two wavelengths work together to target both surface inflammation and deeper joint or muscle issues, leading to quicker relief and healing.
   - **Wound Healing**: For chronic wounds, ulcers, or surgical recovery, the combination can

promote faster cell regeneration at all layers of tissue, supporting the healing process in both surface and deeper tissue layers.

By integrating near-infrared light into the red light therapy routine, individuals can target more complex issues, increase the effectiveness of their therapy, and achieve a broader scope of healing.

Combining with Cold Therapy, Sauna, and Other Modalities

Incorporating other therapeutic modalities alongside red light therapy can significantly enhance results, especially for those dealing with chronic pain, inflammation, muscle recovery, or detoxification. The synergistic effects of combining red light therapy with other treatments can provide a holistic approach to healing and well-being. Here are some popular modalities that work well with red light therapy:

1. **Cold Therapy (Cryotherapy)**
   - **How It Works**: Cryotherapy involves exposing the body or specific areas to extremely cold temperatures, which causes blood vessels to constrict and reduces inflammation. This is especially beneficial for muscle recovery, pain management, and inflammation reduction.
   - **Synergy with Red Light Therapy**: After a cryotherapy session, using red light therapy can promote faster healing by stimulating circulation and enhancing cellular regeneration. Cryotherapy reduces swelling and pain, while red light therapy accelerates tissue repair and regeneration, leading to quicker recovery.
   - **Use Cases**: Athletes and fitness enthusiasts commonly use this combination for post-workout recovery. Individuals with chronic

pain conditions like arthritis or fibromyalgia may also find this combination effective in managing pain and reducing stiffness.

2. **Sauna Therapy**
    - **How It Works**: Infrared saunas work by emitting infrared light that heats the body directly, promoting detoxification, relaxation, improved circulation, and overall well-being. Traditional saunas use heat to induce sweating, which helps detoxify the body.
    - **Synergy with Red Light Therapy**: Combining sauna use with red light therapy takes advantage of both treatments' ability to improve circulation, enhance metabolic processes, and promote muscle recovery. While the sauna promotes sweating and detoxification, red light therapy can help reduce inflammation, repair tissues, and increase energy production in cells.

- **Use Cases**: This combination is ideal for individuals looking to detoxify, reduce muscle soreness, or improve skin health. It is particularly effective for those experiencing chronic pain, tension, or conditions like arthritis, as both therapies work together to reduce inflammation and promote healing.

3. **Massage Therapy**
    - **How It Works**: Massage therapy helps relax muscles, release tension, improve circulation, and promote overall relaxation.
    - **Synergy with Red Light Therapy**: Combining massage with red light therapy can enhance muscle recovery by improving blood flow, reducing muscle soreness, and accelerating tissue healing. The massage helps release built-up toxins and tension in muscles, while red light therapy speeds up the recovery and healing process.

4. **Stretching and Yoga**
    - **How It Works**: Stretching and yoga are excellent for improving flexibility, muscle strength, and joint mobility.
    - **Synergy with Red Light Therapy**: Red light therapy can be used before or after stretching and yoga sessions to reduce inflammation, alleviate muscle stiffness, and enhance recovery. It can also help improve flexibility by promoting increased blood flow to the muscles and tissues being stretched.

Addressing Complex Health Conditions with Red Light Therapy

While red light therapy is commonly used for skin care, muscle recovery, and pain management, its potential extends far beyond these applications. It has been increasingly studied for its impact on more complex health conditions. Let's explore how red light therapy can address some of these challenging conditions:

1. **Neurological Disorders**
    - Red light therapy has shown promise in the treatment of neurological conditions like **Parkinson's disease, Alzheimer's disease**, and **multiple sclerosis**. Near-infrared light can stimulate brain cells and increase mitochondrial activity, which may slow down the progression of these diseases and help preserve cognitive function. Research suggests that red light therapy may also reduce inflammation and oxidative stress in the brain, two major contributors to neurodegenerative diseases.
    - **Use Cases**: People with early-stage Alzheimer's disease may benefit from cognitive improvements when

combining red light therapy with other treatments like physical therapy or memory exercises.
2. **Chronic Pain and Inflammatory Conditions**
    - For conditions like **fibromyalgia**, **rheumatoid arthritis**, and **chronic back pain**, red light therapy is a promising alternative to traditional pain management methods. Its ability to reduce inflammation, promote circulation, and accelerate tissue repair makes it an ideal treatment for managing chronic pain.
    - **Use Cases**: Individuals suffering from autoimmune diseases or fibromyalgia may experience a reduction in pain and inflammation by regularly incorporating red light therapy into their routine.
3. **Mood Disorders**
    - Red light therapy has shown potential in improving symptoms of

mood disorders like **depression** and **seasonal affective disorder (SAD)**. Exposure to light has long been known to influence mood and mental health. Red light therapy, in particular, has been found to stimulate the production of **serotonin**, a neurotransmitter that regulates mood and reduces feelings of anxiety and depression.
- **Use Cases**: People struggling with depression or anxiety, particularly those affected by seasonal changes, may find relief through regular exposure to red light therapy.

4. **Hormonal Imbalances**
   - Red light therapy has been studied for its impact on **hormonal regulation**. It has shown potential in balancing **thyroid hormones**, improving insulin sensitivity, and enhancing **testosterone production**. By stimulating the mitochondria in cells, red light

therapy can help optimise metabolic processes and hormonal function.
- **Use Cases**: Individuals with thyroid imbalances, insulin resistance, or hormonal dysregulation may benefit from red light therapy, either as a primary treatment or as an adjunct to traditional therapies.

Emerging Trends and Experimental Applications

Red light therapy is continuously evolving, with new research exploring its applications in various fields of medicine and wellness. Some of the emerging trends and experimental applications of red light therapy include:

1. **Cancer Treatment**: While red light therapy cannot cure cancer, it is being explored as a complementary treatment to reduce side effects of cancer treatments like chemotherapy and radiation. Red light

therapy may help reduce inflammation, manage pain, and accelerate healing in tissues damaged by cancer treatments.
2. **Hair Restoration**: Red light therapy has shown promise in stimulating hair growth, especially for individuals suffering from **androgenic alopecia (male or female pattern baldness)**. The therapy works by increasing blood circulation to the scalp, stimulating hair follicles, and promoting hair regrowth.
3. **Gene Therapy**: There is growing interest in using red light therapy in combination with gene therapy to enhance cell regeneration and repair. By boosting mitochondrial function and cellular energy, red light therapy may help optimise the delivery and effectiveness of gene therapies.
4. **Sports Medicine**: Red light therapy is becoming increasingly popular in professional sports for enhancing performance, speeding up recovery, and preventing injuries. The integration of red

light therapy with athletic training regimens is a key area of focus in experimental applications, with many athletes reporting significant improvements in performance and recovery times.

Frequently Asked Questions About Red Light Therapy

Red Light Therapy (RLT) is gaining popularity for its wide-ranging benefits, from promoting skin health and muscle recovery to improving mood and cognitive function. Despite its growing use, many people still have questions about how RLT works, its safety, and its effectiveness.

Addressing Common Concerns and Safety Queries

1. **Is Red Light Therapy Safe?** Red light therapy is generally considered safe when used properly. It is a non-invasive, drug-free treatment that has been extensively researched for its ability to stimulate cell regeneration, reduce inflammation, and promote healing. When used according to the manufacturer's instructions, there are minimal risks associated with RLT.
   Safety Tips:
   - **Avoid direct eye exposure**: While red light is not harmful to the eyes in the short term, prolonged exposure to bright light can strain the eyes. It's recommended to wear protective goggles when using high-intensity devices near the face.
   - **Use appropriate devices**: Ensure you are using a device that has been approved for your intended use

(e.g., skin treatment, muscle recovery). Always choose FDA-cleared or medically certified devices for the safest results.
- **Follow usage guidelines**: Adhere to the recommended treatment times, intensity levels, and frequency as outlined by the manufacturer or a healthcare provider. Overuse can lead to skin irritation or discomfort.

2. **Can I Overdo Red Light Therapy?**
While red light therapy is considered very safe, overuse can result in temporary redness or irritation of the skin. It's essential to follow the suggested frequency and duration. For most people, treatments typically last between 10-20 minutes per session, 2-3 times per week. If you experience skin irritation or discomfort, reduce the treatment frequency or consult a healthcare provider.

3. **Are There Any Side Effects?** Side effects from red light therapy are rare and usually mild. Some potential side effects include:
   - Temporary redness or warmth on the skin (similar to the feeling after a mild sunburn).
   - Mild eye irritation if not using protective goggles.
   - Lightheadedness or headache (this can occur if using very high-intensity devices for extended periods).
4. These side effects typically subside shortly after the session. However, if they persist, it is important to consult with a healthcare provider.

Troubleshooting Tips for Optimal Outcomes

1. **Why Am I Not Seeing Results?** There are several factors that could impact the effectiveness of red light therapy:

- **Inconsistent Use**: Results may take time to manifest. It's important to use red light therapy regularly, as suggested, to see long-term benefits. Be patient, as changes such as reduced inflammation, improved skin texture, or pain relief can take several weeks to months.
- **Improper Device Placement**: Make sure the device is positioned at the recommended distance from the skin (typically 6-12 inches). If the device is too far away, the light may not be effective enough. Conversely, being too close can cause discomfort or eye strain.
- **Insufficient Treatment Time**: If you are not adhering to the recommended treatment duration (usually 10-20 minutes per session), you might not be receiving the full benefit. Ensure you are spending enough time with the light on the targeted area.

- **Inadequate Device Quality**: Not all red light devices are created equal. Make sure that you are using a high-quality device with the proper wavelength (600–650 nm for red light and 800–1,100 nm for near-infrared light) for optimal outcomes.

2. **How Long Does It Take to See Results?**
The time frame for seeing visible results depends on the condition being treated:
    - **Skin conditions (wrinkles, acne)**: Some individuals may start seeing improvements within 2-4 weeks, especially for superficial skin conditions. Deeper skin concerns, like wrinkles or scarring, may take longer.
    - **Pain and inflammation**: Individuals using RLT for pain management or muscle recovery may feel relief after a few sessions, but ongoing use is often needed for long-term benefits.

- **Hair growth**: Results for hair restoration can take several months, and consistency is key. Clinical studies suggest that 12-24 weeks of treatment are typically required to notice significant improvements in hair density.

Understanding Contraindications and When to Consult a Doctor

1. **Who Should Avoid Red Light Therapy?** While red light therapy is generally safe for most individuals, there are some contraindications and conditions where caution is advised:
   - **Pregnancy**: Red light therapy is generally considered safe, but it is recommended to avoid use over the abdomen during pregnancy, as there is limited research on its effects during this time.

- **Photosensitivity**: People who are sensitive to light or are on medication that increases sensitivity to light should avoid red light therapy or consult a doctor before use.
- **Certain Eye Conditions**: Individuals with eye diseases like retinopathy or other serious eye conditions should avoid using red light devices that shine directly into the eyes, as this may cause discomfort or worsen symptoms.
- **Cancer patients undergoing chemotherapy**: While RLT can be used to alleviate symptoms like pain, it should be done with caution. Always consult with your oncologist before starting RLT, as its effect on certain cancer treatments is still under research.
- **Active infections**: If you have an active infection, especially on the skin, red light therapy should be

avoided until the infection is treated, as it can sometimes stimulate cellular growth that may aggravate certain conditions.
2. **When Should I Consult a Doctor?** It's essential to consult a healthcare provider if:
    - You have a medical condition that might interact with light therapy (such as photosensitivity, lupus, or skin cancer).
    - You are unsure if RLT is right for your condition.
    - You experience side effects like persistent redness, swelling, or irritation after using the device.
    - You are taking medications that may make you more sensitive to light (such as antibiotics, antidepressants, or certain acne treatments).

Myths vs. Facts: Answering Popular Questions

1. **Myth: Red Light Therapy Is Just Like a Tanning Bed**
     - **Fact**: Red light therapy uses specific wavelengths of light that are non-UV and do not cause tanning or sunburn. Unlike tanning beds, which emit harmful UV rays that can damage the skin, red light therapy stimulates the body's cells without causing harm to the skin.
2. **Myth: Red Light Therapy Works Immediately and Always**
     - **Fact**: While some people experience immediate relief or results after a session, red light therapy generally works best with consistent use over time. Results can vary depending on the condition being treated, and it may take weeks or months to see noticeable improvements.

3. **Myth: All Red Light Devices Are the Same**
    - **Fact**: Not all red light devices are equally effective. It's essential to choose a device with the right light wavelength (around 600–650 nm for red light) and an adequate intensity level (measured in milliwatts per square centimetre, or mW/cm²). Always look for devices that have been tested for safety and efficacy.
4. **Myth: Red Light Therapy Is Only for Skin Care**
    - **Fact**: While red light therapy is highly effective for skin conditions like acne and wrinkles, it can also be used for muscle recovery, pain management, cognitive enhancement, and even hair restoration. Its benefits extend well beyond aesthetics, offering a range of therapeutic applications.

5. **Myth: Red Light Therapy Is Expensive and Only Available in Clinics**
    - **Fact**: Red light therapy has become more affordable, with high-quality devices now available for home use. Devices range from handheld models to full-body panels, offering a range of prices. Home treatments are a cost-effective alternative to expensive clinic sessions.

Real Stories and Testimonials: The Impact of Red Light Therapy on Lives

Red Light Therapy (RLT) has garnered attention worldwide for its remarkable benefits, and numerous individuals have experienced life-changing results. While scientific research supports the effectiveness of RLT, real stories from users offer invaluable insight into the everyday impact of this therapy. Below, we explore success stories from people around the world, showcasing how RLT has transformed lives in a variety of ways. These authentic, relatable testimonials demonstrate the versatility of RLT in addressing pain management, skin rejuvenation, muscle recovery, and mental health.

Success Stories from Users Around the World

1. **Sarah, 42, California – Overcoming Chronic Pain and Boosting Energy** For years, Sarah struggled with chronic pain in her lower back due to a herniated disc. She had tried countless treatments, including physical therapy, pain medications, and even acupuncture, but nothing seemed to provide lasting relief. A friend recommended Red Light Therapy, and while Sarah was initially sceptical, she decided to give it a try. After using a home-based red light device for about 15 minutes a day, five days a week, Sarah began to notice

improvements within two weeks. "I felt an immediate difference in my pain levels, like the deep muscle ache I had lived with for years was starting to fade," she shared. "The energy boost was incredible too. I felt more energised throughout the day, and I was sleeping better at night. I could finally get through the day without relying on painkillers."

After six months of regular use, Sarah reported a significant reduction in back pain, along with better mobility and flexibility. "Red Light Therapy has truly given me my life back. I'm now able to work out, take long walks, and enjoy time with my family without being held back by pain. I honestly feel like a new person."

2. **James, 34, United Kingdom – Healing Sports Injuries Faster** James, an amateur athlete, had been dealing with a recurring hamstring injury that sidelined his passion for running. The constant strain and discomfort led to multiple visits to

Healing With Red Light Therapy

physical therapists, but his recovery was slow and the injury often flared up after intense workouts. James learned about Red Light Therapy from a fellow athlete at the gym who swore by its benefits for muscle recovery.

He decided to invest in a red light therapy panel and began using it after each workout. "Within just a couple of sessions, I noticed a difference in how my muscles felt post-training," James recalled. "There was less soreness, and I was able to recover faster. Over the next few weeks, I felt my hamstring becoming stronger, and I was able to push myself harder without pain. What's more, my overall muscle tone improved, and I didn't experience the same fatigue I used to after runs."

James now uses red light therapy as part of his regular post-workout routine, and his hamstring injury has not recurred. "It has completely transformed how I train and recover. Red Light Therapy isn't just for injury recovery—it's become an essential part of my fitness regimen."

3. **Maria, 60, Spain – Skin Rejuvenation and Anti-Aging Benefits** After years of sun exposure and stress, Maria noticed the signs of ageing were becoming more prominent on her skin, particularly fine lines and wrinkles around her eyes and mouth. As a firm believer in holistic health, she was looking for a non-invasive solution to rejuvenate her skin without resorting to expensive treatments like Botox or facelifts. She turned to Red Light Therapy after reading about its benefits for skin health.

Maria started with a hand-held device, using it daily for 10-15 minutes on her face. "At first, I didn't expect drastic results, but after about a month, I started noticing my skin looking smoother and more radiant. My fine lines softened, and there was a noticeable improvement in skin elasticity," she said. "Now, after six months, the difference is remarkable.

People often comment on how youthful my skin looks, and I feel so much more confident."

What Maria loved most was that the results were gradual and natural-looking. "I wasn't looking for an overnight transformation, but Red Light Therapy has been amazing. I'm not worried about wrinkles anymore. It's a huge confidence booster, and I don't have to worry about harsh chemicals or needles. My skin feels healthier, and the glow is back."

4. **David, 28, Australia – Overcoming Seasonal Depression and Improving Mood** David had long struggled with Seasonal Affective Disorder (SAD), experiencing bouts of deep depression, fatigue, and a lack of motivation during the winter months. The lack of sunlight during the colder months made it even worse, and despite trying therapy and medication, his symptoms persisted. A friend suggested trying Red Light Therapy as a potential mood booster, especially

during the long winter.

David began using a red light panel for 15 minutes each morning, exposing himself to the light during the darkest hours of the day. After just a couple of weeks, he noticed a significant improvement in his mood. "It was like the fog started to lift. I wasn't feeling as sluggish, and I had more energy to get through the day. I even noticed my sleep patterns were improving. I felt like I could actually tackle tasks and get out of bed in the morning without feeling overwhelmed," he said.

After a few months of consistent use, David felt more balanced and in control of his mental health. "It's been life-changing. During the darkest days of winter, Red Light Therapy has given me the energy and motivation to stay productive and positive. I'm no longer confined by the weather and my seasonal blues."

5. **Linda, 50, Canada – Managing Chronic Skin Conditions** Linda had suffered from psoriasis for years, with flare-ups that

affected her scalp, elbows, and knees. The constant itching and discomfort were difficult to manage, and over-the-counter creams and prescriptions never seemed to provide lasting relief. She was looking for alternative solutions and decided to try Red Light Therapy after reading about its anti-inflammatory effects.

Linda used a red light panel on her problem areas every evening for 15 minutes. "Within the first two weeks, I noticed a reduction in redness and irritation. The itchiness wasn't as constant, and the plaques on my skin started to fade," she said. "It wasn't a miracle cure, but after consistent use for three months, I saw a significant improvement. The skin on my elbows and knees became smoother, and the lesions on my scalp were almost gone."

Linda now uses red light therapy as part of her daily routine, and the psoriasis has become much more manageable. "I feel so much better in my skin now. Red Light

Therapy has helped me regain control over my condition, and I'm so glad I found a non-invasive, effective solution."

How Red Light Therapy Has Changed Lives

From reducing chronic pain and speeding up muscle recovery to enhancing skin health and improving mental clarity, Red Light Therapy has helped people from all walks of life live better, healthier lives. The experiences shared by Sarah, James, Maria, David, and Linda demonstrate the broad potential of RLT to improve quality of life and help individuals achieve their health and wellness goals.

In particular, RLT offers a non-invasive, drug-free solution to many chronic conditions. Whether it's reducing chronic pain, rejuvenating the skin, enhancing mood, or speeding up recovery from injuries, users are experiencing significant improvements in their daily lives.

Lessons Learned and Key Takeaways from User Experiences

1. **Consistency is Key**: Many users found that consistent, long-term use of Red Light Therapy was essential to achieving noticeable results. Patience and regular use often led to the most impactful outcomes.
2. **Red Light Therapy is Versatile**: From pain relief and muscle recovery to improving skin health and mental well-being, RLT can be beneficial for a wide range of health conditions, making it a valuable addition to various wellness routines.
3. **Personalised Protocols**: Each individual's experience with Red Light Therapy is unique, and personalised treatment protocols (such as treatment duration, frequency, and device type) can greatly affect the results. Listening to one's body and adjusting accordingly is vital.

4. **The Importance of Quality Devices**: Many users emphasised the importance of investing in a high-quality, properly calibrated device to ensure the most effective outcomes. It's crucial to choose FDA-approved or clinically tested devices for safety and efficacy.
5. **A Complementary Approach**: Many users found that combining Red Light Therapy with other healthy habits, such as exercise, good nutrition, and a healthy sleep routine, significantly amplified the therapy's results.

The Future of Red Light Therapy in Medicine

Red Light Therapy (RLT) has been increasingly recognized as a valuable non-invasive treatment in the field of medicine. Originally used for skin care and wound healing, its applications have expanded across a variety of health conditions, including chronic pain, mental health, muscle recovery, and even cognitive function. As research continues to evolve, so does our understanding of the potential of red and near-infrared light in promoting health and well-being. The future of RLT in medicine looks promising, with new research, emerging technologies, and broader adoption in mainstream and integrative medicine.

New Research and Potential Health Applications

The scientific community is rapidly uncovering new ways that Red Light Therapy can benefit health, and this research is pushing the boundaries of how RLT can be used in medical practice. Several exciting areas of research are already showing promise for future applications:

1. **Neurodegenerative Diseases**: Recent studies suggest that red and near-infrared light may have neuroprotective effects that could slow the progression of neurodegenerative diseases such as Alzheimer's, Parkinson's, and Multiple Sclerosis. Researchers have found that RLT can stimulate mitochondrial function in brain cells, enhance cellular metabolism, and potentially reduce the

harmful buildup of beta-amyloid plaques, a hallmark of Alzheimer's disease. Ongoing trials are testing RLT as a treatment to improve cognitive function and slow down neurodegeneration.
2. **Cancer Treatment**: One of the most exciting and controversial areas of RLT research is its potential role in cancer treatment. Preliminary studies indicate that red light may help to shrink tumours and reduce side effects caused by conventional cancer treatments like chemotherapy and radiation. This effect is believed to be linked to the enhancement of cellular metabolism and the activation of mitochondrial processes. While more research is needed, early results are prompting researchers to explore red light therapy as an adjunct to traditional cancer therapies.
3. **Diabetes and Metabolic Health**: Another promising area of RLT research involves its use in managing metabolic diseases such as diabetes. RLT has been shown to

help reduce inflammation and improve insulin sensitivity, both of which are key factors in the management of Type 2 diabetes. Additionally, studies have shown that RLT can enhance adipose (fat) tissue metabolism, possibly offering a novel approach for managing obesity and metabolic syndrome.

4. **Chronic Inflammatory Conditions**: Red Light Therapy has long been used to reduce inflammation in conditions like arthritis, but new research is expanding its potential applications to other chronic inflammatory diseases, such as Crohn's disease, ulcerative colitis, and fibromyalgia. RLT is being studied for its ability to modulate immune system responses, reduce chronic inflammation, and accelerate tissue repair, making it a promising treatment for a wide range of autoimmune and inflammatory conditions.

5. **Mental Health and Brain Function**: The neurostimulation effects of red light are not limited to neurodegenerative diseases.

In the realm of mental health, RLT has shown promise as a treatment for depression, anxiety, and post-traumatic stress disorder (PTSD). Researchers are particularly interested in how light therapy can affect serotonin production, blood flow to the brain, and overall brainwave activity. Some studies suggest that red light can enhance cognitive performance, alleviate symptoms of depression, and improve focus and mental clarity.

Innovations in Light Therapy Devices and Technologies

As research into Red Light Therapy continues, so do the innovations in light therapy devices and technologies. Several advancements are helping to expand the availability, effectiveness, and accessibility of RLT for both medical and personal use.

1. **Portable and Wearable Devices**: One of the biggest innovations in RLT is the development of portable, easy-to-use devices that can be used at home or on the go. Wearable devices, such as light-emitting patches, caps, and gloves, are enabling users to target specific areas of the body without being restricted to a clinic or treatment centre. These devices offer the convenience of at-home therapy, making RLT more accessible to those who need it most.

2. **More Targeted and Personalised Treatment**: Recent advancements in RLT devices have allowed for more precise control of light intensity, wavelength, and exposure time, making treatment protocols more personalised. Devices can now be tailored to address specific conditions such as skin care, muscle recovery, or even cognitive function. With the integration of AI and machine learning, devices may soon be able to track a user's response to treatment and

automatically adjust settings for optimal results.

3. **Combination Devices**: Innovations in combination therapies are also on the rise, where red light is combined with other modalities like infrared light, heat therapy, or even microcurrent stimulation. These combination devices are designed to enhance the effectiveness of RLT by addressing multiple therapeutic needs at once. For example, combining red light therapy with heat therapy can stimulate increased blood flow, improving the delivery of oxygen and nutrients to tissues.

4. **Clinical-Grade Light Therapy Equipment**: While at-home devices are becoming more widespread, the development of advanced clinical-grade equipment continues to push the boundaries of medical use for RLT. High-powered devices used in clinical settings are increasingly designed for more complex conditions such as deep

tissue injuries, joint regeneration, and even cancer therapies. These devices often employ larger panels or full-body light beds, providing patients with intensive light exposure for maximum therapeutic effects.

Red Light Therapy in Mainstream and Integrative Medicine

As Red Light Therapy gains more recognition and evidence of its therapeutic benefits, it is increasingly being integrated into both mainstream medical practices and alternative health circles. The future of RLT in medicine lies in its ability to complement conventional treatments while also providing a non-invasive, drug-free option for patients.

1. **Integration in Pain Management and Orthopedics**: RLT has been adopted by many physical therapists, chiropractors, and orthopaedic specialists as part of their

pain management protocols. It is commonly used to treat conditions like joint pain, muscle sprains, tendonitis, and arthritis. RLT is seen as an excellent complement to other therapies, such as manual manipulation, heat, and cold therapy, making it a mainstream treatment in the world of physical rehabilitation.

2. **Role in Anti-Aging and Aesthetic Medicine**: Red Light Therapy is already widely used in the field of dermatology and cosmetic surgery. Its ability to rejuvenate the skin, stimulate collagen production, and reduce wrinkles has made it a staple in non-invasive facial treatments. As the demand for non-surgical anti-aging treatments continues to grow, RLT will likely play an even larger role in aesthetics and beauty treatments.

3. **Holistic and Integrative Health Practices**: Beyond conventional medicine, RLT is gaining traction in holistic and integrative health practices. Wellness

practitioners often combine RLT with acupuncture, herbal therapies, massage, and other natural treatments to promote healing and balance in the body. This integrated approach offers patients a comprehensive, non-pharmaceutical solution to a variety of health issues, from chronic pain to mental health challenges.

4. **Sports Medicine and Athletic Performance**: The use of Red Light Therapy in sports medicine is expected to increase, particularly for injury recovery and performance enhancement. RLT's ability to accelerate tissue repair and reduce inflammation makes it an essential tool in the rehabilitation of athletes. Professional athletes are already incorporating RLT into their recovery routines, and it is expected that more sports teams and clinics will adopt this technology in the future.

How Red Light Therapy Is Shaping the Future of Wellness

Red Light Therapy is not only revolutionising medical treatments but also reshaping the future of wellness. With its versatility, non-invasive nature, and growing body of research, RLT is positioned to become a mainstream wellness tool that people can use to improve their health and vitality.

1. **Accessibility and Affordability**: As RLT devices become more affordable and accessible, they are poised to become a staple in households across the globe. With wearable and portable devices now on the market, people can easily incorporate RLT into their daily wellness routines. The growing trend of self-care and prevention will likely drive further adoption of RLT as an everyday wellness tool.
2. **Preventative Healthcare**: One of the most exciting developments in the future of Red Light Therapy is its potential in

preventive healthcare. By promoting cellular health, reducing inflammation, and improving circulation, RLT can help prevent a wide range of conditions before they become chronic. This preventive approach aligns with the increasing emphasis on maintaining wellness rather than just treating illness, a trend that will likely shape the future of healthcare in general.

3. **Integrating with Personalized Health Programs**: The future of RLT will likely involve its integration into personalised health and wellness programs. Advances in genetic testing, wearable health technology, and data analytics are helping to create customised health plans for individuals. Red Light Therapy will be an important tool in these programs, offering patients a tailored, evidence-based solution for improving their health outcomes.

Appendices

In this section, we provide additional resources, references, and definitions to enhance your understanding of Red Light Therapy (RLT) and its applications. This appendix includes a **Glossary of Terms and Scientific Concepts**, **Recommended Red Light Therapy Resources and Products**, and **Key Research Studies and References** to serve as valuable resources for anyone exploring or utilising RLT for health and wellness.

Glossary of Terms and Scientific Concepts

A thorough understanding of the scientific principles behind Red Light Therapy (RLT) can help you make the most of this therapy. Below is a glossary of key terms and concepts related to RLT, which can provide clarity when navigating the technical aspects of light therapy.

1. Light Wavelength: The distance between two peaks of a light wave, measured in nanometers (nm). Different wavelengths of light can penetrate the skin to varying depths and affect tissues differently. Red light typically ranges from 600-650 nm, while near-infrared light falls between 700-1,100 nm.

2. Mitochondria: The powerhouses of cells that generate energy in the form of ATP (adenosine triphosphate). Red Light Therapy helps stimulate mitochondrial activity, leading to increased ATP production, which aids in cellular repair and regeneration.

3. ATP (Adenosine Triphosphate): A molecule that provides energy for cellular processes. By increasing ATP production, Red Light Therapy accelerates healing, reduces inflammation, and promotes overall cell function.

4. Photobiomodulation (PBM): A process where light photons are absorbed by cells, stimulating biological processes. PBM is the underlying mechanism of action for Red Light Therapy, promoting healing, reducing pain, and improving tissue regeneration.

5. Chromophores: Molecules within cells that absorb specific wavelengths of light. In RLT, chromophores in the mitochondria and other cell components absorb light energy to enhance cellular function and repair.

6. Haemoglobin and Myoglobin: Oxygen-carrying proteins found in the blood and muscles, respectively. RLT helps improve oxygen delivery to tissues by increasing blood flow and the absorption of oxygen in these proteins.

7. Inflammation: A natural immune response to injury or infection, but when chronic, it can lead to tissue damage and various diseases. Red Light Therapy helps reduce inflammation, promoting faster healing and relieving pain.

8. Collagen: A protein that provides structure to the skin, tendons, ligaments, and bones. RLT has been shown to stimulate collagen production, contributing to skin rejuvenation, wound healing, and joint health.

9. Near-Infrared Light (NIR): A type of light that is invisible to the naked eye but can penetrate deep into tissues, promoting healing and reducing pain. NIR is often used in combination with red light for a broader range of therapeutic benefits.

10. Wavelength Spectrum: The range of wavelengths that light can travel in, from visible light to infrared. Red Light Therapy typically utilises the red and near-infrared parts of the spectrum for its therapeutic effects.

11. Photoreceptors: Cellular structures that absorb light energy and trigger biological responses. In the case of RLT, photoreceptors in the mitochondria and cell membranes are activated by specific wavelengths of light, promoting healing.

12. Vasodilation: The widening of blood vessels, which increases blood flow to tissues. RLT can induce vasodilation, leading to better oxygen and nutrient delivery, which enhances the healing process.

13. Neuroprotection: The process of protecting neurons from injury or degeneration. Some studies suggest that RLT may have neuroprotective effects that could benefit patients with neurodegenerative diseases such as Alzheimer's and Parkinson's.

14. Hyperpigmentation: The darkening of the skin due to excess melanin. Red Light Therapy has been shown to help reduce hyperpigmentation by promoting healthy skin cell turnover and collagen production.

15. Oxidative Stress: An imbalance between free radicals and antioxidants in the body. RLT helps mitigate oxidative stress, which plays a role in ageing and various chronic diseases.

Recommended Red Light Therapy Resources and Products

For those looking to explore Red Light Therapy in more depth or invest in devices for personal use, the following resources and products come highly recommended. They offer valuable insights into RLT and provide effective devices for a range of therapeutic needs.

Books

1. **"The Red Light Therapy Bible" by Kate Dawson**
   This comprehensive guide covers the science behind RLT, practical tips for treatment, and a deep dive into its applications for skin health, pain management, and muscle recovery.
2. **"Healing Light: Red Light Therapy for Wellness" by Dr. Melissa Cassidy**
   This book is ideal for those looking to incorporate RLT into their daily wellness routines. Dr. Cassidy provides an accessible breakdown of the benefits and

how RLT can improve sleep, mental health, and overall well-being.
3. **"Photobiomodulation in the Brain: Clinical Effects and Mechanisms" by Dr. Michael R. Hamblin**
For those interested in the neuroprotective effects of RLT, this book provides detailed scientific research on how red light and near-infrared light can enhance brain health and cognitive function.

Devices

1. **Joovv Red Light Therapy Devices**
Joovv is a popular brand in the red light therapy space, offering full-body panels and targeted handheld devices that provide both red and near-infrared light for therapeutic benefits. Their devices are clinically proven and highly rated by users for their quality and effectiveness.
2. **Red Light Man**
Known for producing high-quality red light therapy devices, Red Light Man offers a range of products, from small

handheld devices for targeted treatments to larger panels for full-body exposure. Their devices are optimised for clinical use and home treatments.

3. **Mito Red Light**
   Mito Red Light is another top brand offering affordable yet effective red light therapy products, ranging from portable units to high-powered panels. Their devices are known for their customizable settings and ease of use.

4. **Therabody Theragun**
   While not a traditional red light therapy device, the Theragun is a percussive therapy tool that complements light therapy treatments by targeting muscle soreness and improving circulation, making it a great addition to a holistic recovery routine.

5. **LightStim for Pain**
   This FDA-approved handheld device uses LED light therapy to reduce pain and inflammation. It's a great option for individuals seeking targeted pain relief for

conditions like arthritis, muscle strains, and joint pain.

Key Research Studies and References

Here are some key research studies and references that offer in-depth scientific insights into the mechanisms and effectiveness of Red Light Therapy.

1. **Hamblin, M. R. (2017). "Photobiomodulation or Low-Level Laser Therapy."** *Journal of Biophotonics, 10(12), 978-994.*
   This study provides a comprehensive review of the biological mechanisms behind photobiomodulation and its therapeutic effects. It explains how light interacts with cells to stimulate healing and reduce inflammation.
2. **Cerniglia, L., & Bibb, D. (2018). "The Use of Red and Near-Infrared Light for Post-Surgical Recovery."** *Journal of*

Surgical Research, 226, 1-8.
This study explores how red and near-infrared light can accelerate recovery after surgery by enhancing mitochondrial function, improving circulation, and reducing pain and inflammation.

3. Naeser, M. A., et al. (2011). "Improvement of Cognitive Function and Mood in Patients with Traumatic Brain Injury Using Near-Infrared Light." *Journal of Neurotrauma, 28*(2), 227-234.
This research investigates the potential of near-infrared light therapy in improving cognitive function in patients with brain injuries. It highlights the neuroprotective benefits and potential applications in cognitive rehabilitation.

4. Tuner, J., & Hode, L. (2004). "The Laser Therapy Handbook: A Practical Guide to the Therapeutic Use of Light." *Medical Laser Applications, 19*(4), 41-45.
This handbook is a valuable resource for those seeking to understand the

therapeutic uses of lasers and light in various medical applications, including wound healing, pain management, and skin rejuvenation.

5. **Zhao, S. T., & Zhang, X. J. (2015). "Effects of Low-Level Laser Therapy on Muscle Healing."** *European Journal of Physiology, 467*(3), 497-506.
This study evaluates the effects of low-level laser therapy (LLLT), including red light, on muscle tissue repair. It demonstrates how light therapy can enhance muscle recovery, reduce soreness, and speed up healing.

6. **Litscher, G., et al. (2014). "Use of Laser and Light in Medicine: From Mechanisms to Practical Applications."** *Lasers in Surgery and Medicine, 46*(1), 34-40.
This article provides an in-depth review of the current research on laser and light therapies, covering a broad range of medical applications from skin care to pain management.

Healing With Red Light Therapy

Healing With Red Light Therapy

www.ingramcontent.com/pod-product-compliance
Lightning Source LLC
Chambersburg PA
CBHW070421240526
45472CB00019B/88